Neural Control of the Semispinalis Cervicis Muscle and the Influence of Neck Pain

Neural Control of the Semispinalis Cervicis Muscle and the Influence of Neck Pain

PhD Thesis by

Jochen Schomacher

*Center for Sensory-Motor Interaction (SMI),
Department of Health Science and Technology,
Aalborg University, Aalborg, Denmark*

River Publishers

Aalborg

ISBN 978-87-92982-20-9 (paperback)
ISBN 978-87-92982-19-3 (e-book)

Published, sold and distributed by:
River Publishers
P.O. Box 1657
Algade 42
9000 Aalborg
Denmark

Tel.: +45369953197
www.riverpublishers.com

Table of contents

Abstract

The objective of this thesis was to investigate the activation of a deep cervical extensor, the semispinalis cervicis, in asymptomatic individuals and patients with neck pain. Together with the deep flexor muscles the deep cervical extensors contribute to support and stabilization of the cervical spine. Impaired activation of these muscles may contribute to the recurrence and maintenance of neck pain and consequently assessing and restoring the function of the deep muscles is considered to be important in the rehabilitation of patients with neck pain. Preliminary evidence for lower activation of the deep cervical extensors in patients with neck pain was shown in only one study which utilized functional magnetic resonance imaging (MRI) to evaluate the activation of the deep muscles. This thesis directly examined the neural control of the semispinalis cervicis using ultrasound guided intramuscular electromyography (EMG) and compared the activation of the semispinalis cervicis in patients with chronic neck pain and in healthy controls. Finally, the possibility of emphasizing the activation of this muscle by specific exercise was evaluated.

Four studies were performed. First, the neural drive to fascicles of the semispinalis cervicis at two different spinal levels was investigated in healthy subjects in order to examine whether all fascicles of the muscle receive common or independent neural drive. In a second study, the activity of semispinalis cervicis was examined in patients with neck pain and compared to healthy controls to examine whether this muscle is activated differently in patients. In the third study the tenderness to pressure of the tissues over the cervical zygapophyseal joints was measured using the pressure pain threshold (PPT) at two spinal levels. Furthermore, the activity of the semispinalis cervicis was measured at the same levels and a correlation analysis was performed between PPT and EMG measures. In the fourth and final study the activation of semispinalis cervicis in relation to the superficial extensor splenius capitis was investigated during three different exercises.

The results showed a lower recruitment threshold and a higher number of active motor units in the fascicle of the semispinalis cervicis at the spinal level C5 compared to C2 reflecting a partially independent neural drive to fascicles of semispinalis cervicis. The independent drive to different fascicles of the muscle may be determined by mechanical needs and advantages of different fascicles for the task performed. The second study of the thesis showed that patients with chronic neck pain display lower activity of the semispinalis cervicis compared to healthy controls. Furthermore, the directional specificity of semispinalis cervicis was lower in patients, i.e. the ability to contract in well-defined preferred directions according to the muscle's anatomical position relative to the spine. In the second study the activation of the semispinalis cervicis muscles was measured at C3. In the third study the activation of semispinalis cervicis muscle was monitored at both C2 and C5 and the results showed that patients with neck pain also display lower and less defined activation of the semispinalis cervicis at these levels suggesting that altered activation of this muscle is generalized to all levels of the cervical spine and is not unique to one spinal level. PPT measured over C2 and C5 correlated significantly, albeit only weakly with EMG amplitude and the directional specificity of semispinalis cervicis when the control and patient data was pooled together, suggesting that other factors like general psychological distress, fear avoidance behavior and disuse may contribute this finding. Finally, the activity of the semispinalis cervicis increased relative to the splenius capitis when the patient pushed dorsally against the therapist's manual resistance at the vertebral arch of C2. This did not occur when pushing backwards against resistance applied at either the occiput or at C5.

Taken together, these findings indicate that the neural control of the semispinalis cervicis muscle is altered in patients with chronic neck pain. Furthermore, patients with the highest pressure pain sensitivity displayed the greatest impairment in activation of the semispinalis cervicis. Given the role of the deep cervical extensors in the provision of support to the cervical spine, impaired control of this muscle may have relevance for the perpetuation or maintenance of neck pain. A specific exercise was shown to increase the activity of semispinalis cervicis relative to the superficial splenius capitis, suggesting that this exercise would be useful to include an exercise program for patients with neck pain. Further research is necessary to investigate the efficacy of such an exercise in patients with neck pain.

Abstrakt

Neural kontrol af m. semispinalis cervicis og indvirkning på nakkesmerter

Formålet med denne afhandling var at undersøge aktiveringen af den dybe nakkeextensor, m. semispinalis cervicis, hos symptomfri personer og patienter med nakkesmerter. Sammen med de dybe fleksormuskler bidrager nakkeextensorerne til støtte og stabilisering af columna cervicalis. Svækket aktivering af disse muskler kan bidrage til gentagne og vedvarende nakkesmerter, og som følge heraf anses vurdering og genopretning af funktionen af de dybe muskler for vigtig i rehabiliteringen af patienter med nakkesmerter. Foreløbig har kun et studie fremlagt bevis for lavere aktivering af de dybe nakkeextensorer. Dette studie anvendte magnetisk resonans billeddannelse (MRI) til at vurdere aktiveringen af de dybe muskler. Denne afhandling har direkte undersøgt den neurale kontrol af m. semispinalis cervicis ved hjælp af ultralydskontrolleret intramuskulær elektromyografi (EMG) og sammenlignede aktivering af m. semispinalis cervicis hos patienter med kroniske nakkesmerter og raske forsøgspersoner. Endvidere blev muligheden for forbedring af aktiveringen af denne muskel ved hjælp af specifikke øvelser vurderet.

Der blev udført fire studier i forbindelse med afhandlingen. I første studie undersøgtes den neurale aktivering til fiberbundter i m. semispinalis cervicis på to forskellige spinale niveauer hos raske forsøgspersoner for at undersøge, om alle fiberbundter i musklen modtager en fælles eller en uafhængig neural aktivering. I det andet studie undersøgtes aktiviteten i m. semispinalis cervicis hos patienter med nakkesmerter, og denne blev herefter sammenlignet med raske forsøgspersoner for at undersøge, om denne muskel aktiveres forskelligt hos patienter. I det tredje studie måltes ømhed for tryk på vævet over de zygapophysiale led ved hjælp af tryksmertetærskler (PPT) på to spinale niveauer. Endvidere måltes aktiviteten af m. semispinalis cervicis på de samme niveauer og der udførtes en korrelationsanalyse mellem PPT og EMG-målinger. I fjerde og sidste studie undersøgtes aktiveringen af m. semispinalis cervicis i relation til overflade-extensoren m. splenius capitis under tre forskellige øvelser.

Resultaterne viste en lavere rekrutteringstærskel og et højere antal aktive motorenheder i m. semispinalis cervicis' fiberbundt på det spinale niveau C5 sammenlignet med C2, hvilket afspejler en delvis uafhængig aktivering til fiberbundterne i m. semispinalis cervicis. Den uafhængige aktivering til forskellige fiberbundter i musklen kan bestemmes af mekaniske behov og fordele ved forskellige fiberbunder til den udførte opgave. Det andet studie viste, at patienter med kroniske nakkesmerter udviser lavere aktivitet i m. semispinalis cervicis sammenlignet med kontrolgruppen. Endvidere var retningspecifiteten af m. semispinalis cervicis lavere hos patienterne, dvs. evnen til sammentrækning i veldefinerede foretrukne retninger i henhold til musklens anatomiske placering i forhold til rygraden. I andet studie måltes aktiveringen af m. semispinalis cervicis ved C3. I det tredje studie blev aktiveringen af m. semispinalis cervicis undersøgt ved både C2 og C5, og resultaterne viste, at patienter med nakkesmerter også udviser lavere og mindre defineret aktivering af m. semispinalis cervicis på disse niveauer, hvilket indikerer, at ændret aktivering af denne muskel kan generaliseres til alle niveauer af columna cervicalis og ikke er unik for ét spinalt niveau. PPT målt over C2 og C5 korrelerede signifikant, om end kun svagt med EMG-amplitude og retningsspecifitet af m. semispinalis cervicis, når data fra kontrolgruppen og patienter blev lagt sammen, hvilket tyder på, at andre faktorer som generelle psykologiske bekymringer, undgåelsesadfærd og misbrug kan bidrage til dette resultat. Endelig blev aktiviteten af m. semispinalis cervicis forøget i forhold til m. splenius capitis, når patienten trykkede dorsalt mod forskerens modstand ved arcus vertebrae C2. Dette skete ikke, når forsøgspersonen skubbede bagover mod modstand påført enten på baghoved eller ved C5.

Alt i alt indikerer disse resultater, at den neurale kontrol af m. semispinalis cervicis ændres hos patienter med kroniske nakkesmerter. Endvidere viste patienterne med den højeste tryksmertefølsomhed den største svækkelse i aktivering af m. semispinalis cervicis. På baggrund af de dybe nakkeextensorers rolle i tilvejebringelsen af støtte til columna cervicalis kan svækket kontrol af denne muskel have relevans for fortsatte nakkesmerter. En specifik øvelse viste sig at forøge aktiviteten af m. semispinalis cervicis i forhold til m. splenius capitis, hvilket indikerer, at denne øvelse kan være brugbar i et program med øvelser til patienter med nakkesmerter. Yderligere forskning er nødvendigt for at undersøge virkningen af denne øvelse hos patienter med nakkesmerter.

Acknowledgments

I would like to thank my supervisor Deborah Falla for accepting my proposal of this project made during a congress the 15th November 2008 in Parma, Italy. Her support and guidance have been essential for completing this thesis. Thanks also to Dario Farina and his team, to René Lindstrøm, Shellie Boudreau, and Jakob Lund Dideriksen. Their help and especially Jakob's EMG knowledge were most valuable!

A great thank you goes to Elio Stella who like a father taught me how to work and to live. Without him this thesis and many other projects wouldn't have been completed! Thanks also to Freddy Kaltenborn who showed me the fascination of physiotherapy revealing its simplicity and logic.

Publications

This thesis is based on the following publications

Study 1:
Schomacher J, Dideriksen J L, Farina D, Falla D. Recruitment of motor units in two fascicles of the semispinalis cervicis muscle. The Journal of Neurophysiology, 2012; 107(11): 3078-3085 / doi: 10.1152/jn.00953.2011.

Study 2:
Schomacher J, Farina D, Lindstroem R, Falla D. Chronic trauma-induced neck pain impairs the neural control of the deep semispinalis cervicis muscle. Clinical Neurophysiology, 123(7), 2012: 1403-1408 / doi: 10.1016/j.clinph.2011.11.033.

Study 3:
Schomacher J, Boudreau S A, Petzke F, Falla D. Localized pain sensitivity is associated with reduced activation of the semispinalis cervicis muscle in patients with neck pain. Clinical Journal of Pain. 2013 Jan 30. [Epub ahead of print]

Study 4:
Schomacher J, Petzke F, Falla D. Localised resistance selectively activates the semispinalis cervicis muscle in patients with neck pain. Manual Therapy, 2012 Dec;17(6):544-548 / doi: 10.1016/j.math.2012.05.012.

Abbreviations

–	AP	action potential	–	MU:	motor unit
–	ARV:	average rectified value	–	MUAP:	motor unit action potential
–	CIS:	Common Input Strength index	–	MUAPT:	motor unit action potential train
–	CSA:	cross-sectional area			
–	EMG:	electromyography	–	N:	Newton
–	Hz:	Hertz	–	pps:	pulses per second
–	iEMG:	intramuscular EMG	–	PPT:	pressure pain threshold
–	ISI:	interspike intervals			
–	kPa:	kilo Pascal	–	RCT:	randomized controlled trial
–	LED:	light-emitting diode			
–	MFAP:	muscle fiber action potential	–	SE:	standard error
–	mfMRI:	muscle functional magnetic resonance imaging			

Overview

„La pazienza vince tutto!" (Elio Stella)
Patience overcomes anything!

Chapter 1 describes the anatomy and function of the cervical muscles and reviews the neuromuscular dysfunctions associated with neck pain.

Chapter 2 explains the neurophysiology of muscle activation and electromyography. This chapter also presents the aims of this thesis.

Chapter 3 describes the common methods used in the thesis.

Chapter 4 reports the results followed by a discussion of each study.

Chapter 5 discusses the main results, considers limitations of the studies and provides suggestions for further research.

Chapter 6 presents a general conclusion of the thesis.

The **appendixes** contain tables showing an overview of the common methods and the main results.

The **references** are listed in this part of the thesis.

Paper 1 to 4 contain the original studies on which this thesis is based.

Chapter 1.

Rationale of the topic

1.1 INTRODUCTION

Neck pain represents a serious suffering for patients and an economic burden for the society [1]. In most cases a structure causing the pain cannot be identified and consequently a reasonable pharmacological or surgical treatment can rarely be offered [2]. Most patients receive conservative treatment and many seek help by physiotherapists [3]. Different treatments have shown efficacy for reducing neck pain like low-level laser therapy [4], a multi-component pain and stress self-management group intervention [5], massage [6], cervical joint mobilization [7, 8], and upper thoracic spine thrust manipulation for reducing pain and improving function [9-12]. Comprehensive literature analyses however do question the efficacy of massage [13] and mobilization [14]. Many studies show efficacy of exercises for reducing neck pain and associated disability [15-17] as also a comprehensive literature review [18]. The best type of exercise however is still unclear [19]. For the cervical flexor group different dysfunctions have been identified like reduced activation of the deep cervical flexors longus capitis and longus colli muscles during a task of cranio-cervical flexion [20]. The superficial flexors like sternocleidomastoid and anterior scalene muscles show concomitantly increased activation [21] aiming probably to maintain cervical stability [20]. Appropriate exercises have shown efficacy in re-establishing a normal activation pattern of superficial and deep cervical flexors [22, 23] and in reducing pain [24, 25] especially in patients having least activation before the training [26]. The cervical extensors are believed to be similarly important for the rehabilitation of patients with neck pain [27]. Knowledge on their activation however is scarce. The general aim of this thesis therefore is to investigate the activation of the deep cervical extensors in healthy subjects and patients with chronic neck pain. Furthermore, the effect of a traditional exercise to increase the activation of the deep cervical extensors in patients with neck pain will be analyzed.

1.2 EPIDEMIOLOGY OF NECK PAIN

Neck pain is a frequent symptom in the world population, more so in women than in men [28]. Life time prevalence of neck pain varies between 43% and 66.7% [29-33]. The prevalence rate in one year varies between 17.9% [34], 53.6% [29] and 64% [1]. With a point prevalence of 22.2% [31] and 20.6% it is the most frequent musculoskeletal complaint after low back and shoulder pain [35]. The differences between the epidemiological studies might be explained by the populations studied and by influencing factors like climate, level of education, means of livelihood and average age of the population [36].

Neck pain is a long-standing problem [37, 38]. Between half and three quarters of patients with neck pain will experience recurrence within 1 to 5 years [39]. Costs for the society due to neck pain are consequently high [40, 41]. Effective treatment of neck pain is therefore needed.

1.3 AETIOLOGY OF NECK PAIN

Neck pain can follow trauma like whiplash, but often the triggering and maintaining causes are unknown [2]. In approximately 80% of patients neck pain is "of unknown origin", that is, idiopathic neck pain [42]. Psychosocial factors like high work demand and job dissatisfaction as well as work-related physical factors are associated with neck pain [43]. There is however no evidence for psychosocial factors being a cause of neck pain [2]. This thesis focuses on the biological aspect of muscle dysfunction related to neck pain.

The biomedical diagnosis of neck pain can be structural and functional. Structures responsible for pain are mainly the intervertebral disc, zygapophyseal joints, muscles, and the neural system. Prevalence for pain originating from the cervical disc ranges between 16 and 41 % [44]. Each cervical disc can provoke well-defined pain patterns in the neck and the adjacent regions including the upper extremities [45]. The diagnosis of disc pain can only be made with discography and is not possible by clinical means alone [2, 44].

The incidence for pain coming from the zygapophyseal joints can be over 60% [46-51]. Also zygapophyseal joint pain can only be diagnosed with invasive means like local anaesthesia [2]. Other possible sources of pain are the (subchondral) bone, and ligaments, which can be injured by for example a whiplash injury [44, 52]. The neural system, for example cervical radiculopathy, is a further possible cause of pain [53]. Again, the clinical diagnosis of these structural causes is difficult.

Muscles can be a primary structural cause of acute neck pain, for example, in an acute muscle sprain [2]. Muscle dysfunction also occurs as a secondary response to pain [2] and may contribute to the maintenance and recurrence of neck pain. For example, alterations in muscle activity may increase stress and the risk of micro-/macrotrauma which can cause and maintain neck pain [2, 54-56].

Experimental pain studies stimulating nociceptors in the muscle confirm that pain can induce immediate changes in neuromuscular control of the neck similar to those observed in patients with neck pain [57, 58]. Furthermore, latent myofascial trigger points are able to change the muscle activation pattern even in the absence of pain [59].

Clinicians like physiotherapists are invited to make a more functional diagnosis before trying to identify the pain provoking structure [60]. When physiotherapists for example find joint dysfunction in the segments C0 to C4, restricted movement in extension and muscle impairment in the cranio-cervcial flexion test, they can distinguish cervicogenic headache from migraine and tension-type headache with a 100% sensitivity and a 94% specificity [61]. Functional findings can correlate with a structural diagnosis: restricted rotation < 60° and positive signs in the upper limb tension test for the median nerve, the neck distraction and the Spurling test for example indicate cervical radiculopathy with a positive likelihood ratio point estimate of 30.3 [53]. Many of these movement changes are an expression of altered motor control which is consequently essential for the understanding of patients with neck pain.

1.4 MOTOR CONTROL OF THE CERVICAL SPINE

Upright relaxed standing body posture is maintained partially by normal passive muscle tone with minimally increased energy costs of ~7% over supine lying [62]. Passive muscle tone is the intrinsic viscoelastic tension provided by passive mechanical properties like inertia, viscosity, and elasticity of muscle tissue [63, 64]. During postural perturbations applied to the trunk the passive muscle tone is supported by co-activation of agonist and antagonist muscles which is considered a normal stabilizing motor strategy in healthy subjects [65]. The importance of muscles is highlighted by the fact that they contribute in vitro to approximately 80% of cervical spine stability [66]. In addition to postural stability of the head the cervical spine has to orient the head with its sensory organs vision, hearing, smelling and balance in the space and in relation to the body [67].

Stability and movement of the spine are controlled by the sensorimotor system which comprises afferent, efferent, and central integration and processing components [68]. The active static and dynamic control of the cervical spine is determined via feedforward and feedback procedures by several mechanisms like voluntary control, proprioception of the neck, and exteroception from the sense organs including the vestibular system [64]. Proprioceptive afferents come probably more from the muscle spindles than from joint receptors [69]. The neck afferents are involved in reflexes which influence head orientation, eye movement control, and postural stability. These reflexes include the cervicocollic reflex (CCR), the cervico-ocular reflex (COR), and the tonic neck reflex (TNR). They work in conjunction with other cervical, vestibular, and visual reflexes acting on the neck musculature [42, 69]. Conflicting afferent information from these systems might contribute to reduced range of movement, pathological movement patterns (reduced acceleration and velocity, reduced smoothness and irregular axes of neck movement), altered intensity and timing of muscle activation, less strength and endurance and problems in maintaining a stable upright posture all of which have been observed in patients with neck pain disorders [70].

1.5 FUNCTIONAL CHANGES IN THE NECK MUSCLES ASSOCIATED WITH PAIN

Neuromuscular adaptations associated with pain are not only a reaction to stimulation of peripheral nociceptors but rather are the result of the interactions between biological, psychological, and social elements of the pain experience [42].

Consequently a number of functional adaptations can be seen in patients with neck pain and these changes will be briefly reviewed below.

1.5.1 Strength

Strength is significantly less in patients with neck pain compared to healthy controls with a large variability ranging from 18 [71] to 90% [72]. Two studies for example reported a loss of overall force of about 29% [73, 74]. These data are coming from cross-sectional studies and consequently we do not know the time course of strength reduction associated with neck pain. Strength tests might rather report the patient's ability to bear strain during the strength test [75] because the average maximum voluntary force of patients with chronic neck pain is inversely and moderately correlated to the pain experienced during the maximal contraction, to fear of movement and to aspects of neck disability like inactivity leading to deconditioning [71].

1.5.2 Endurance

Static endurance of the neck flexors is mostly tested with the maximal holding time in the cervical flexion test, i.e. lifting the head 1 cm from the treatment table keeping the face in the horizontal plane [23, 76]. Several studies have shown a wide range between healthy subjects (14.5 to 95.7 s) and patients with neck pain (16.6 to 24.1 s) indicating however mean values of less endurance in patients with neck pain compared to healthy controls [77, 78]. The test is sufficiently reliable [79]. Endurance of the deep craniocervical flexors is tested with a repeated holding time of minimally 10 s at each stage of the craniocervical flexion test (from 20 to 30 mmHg in steps of 2 mmHg) [42] and also reduced in patients with neck pain [80].

The maximum holding time for the neck extensors is measured in a modified version of the low-back extensor endurance test of Biering-Sørensen [81] in which the prone lying subject holds his head in a horizontal position. The maximum holding time of healthy subjects was with 608.3 s ±39.9 (mean/SD) higher than that of patients with neck pain having sought treatment (350.4 s ± 199.3) and patients without having received treatment yet (480.8 s ±167.8), all differences being statistically significant [82]. The long duration of this test (up to 10 min) however reduces its practicability. The high inter-subject variability of the holding time for the flexors and the extensors questions the clinical value of endurance tests [83]. No literature has been found regarding dynamic endurance, i.e. the maximal repetition number and time of dynamic movements. In addition, myoelectric manifestations of fatigue such as a greater decrease of mean and median frequency has been shown for the sternocleidomastoid and anterior scalene muscles of patients with chronic neck pain compared to matched controls [84]. Greater muscle fatigue was shown ipsilateral to the side of pain in patients with neck pain [85].

1.5.3 Activation strategies

The deep cervical flexors can be activated selectively with the craniocervical flexion movement as shown by EMG [86, 87] and muscle functional MRI [78]. Their activity is lower in patients with neck pain compared to healthy controls [20]. The activity of the superficial flexors like anterior scalene and sternocleidomastoid muscles on the contrary is typically higher in patients with neck pain compared to controls [20, 21, 88]. The EMG activity of the superficial flexors, sternocleidomastoid and anterior scalenes, showed a weak positive correlation with pain intensity during the craniocervical flexion test [89].

During rapid flexion/extension of the arm patients with neck pain presented with delayed onset of activity in the deep cervical flexors, sternocleidomastoid, and the anterior scalene [90]. These muscles were activated within nearly 100 ms for extension and nearly 200 ms for flexion of deltoid onset during rapid arm movements while in healthy subject their activation occurred within 50 ms [90]. The higher the intensity of the patients' pain, the later the onset of activity and lower amplitude of activity of the deep cervical flexors during rapid arm flexion movements [91]. This delayed onset of muscle activity might create non-physiological tissue loading. Some patients also show delayed offset (relaxation) of the sternocleidomastoid muscle[92] and of upper trapezius, cervical extensors and anterior scalene muscles after a repetitive upper limb task [93]. Delayed on- and offset of muscle activity has also been observed for the the sacro-iliac joint [94] and the lumbar spine [95] in patients with chronic low back pain.

The superficial extensors of patients with neck pain showed higher activity during a unilateral upper limb task compared to healthy controls [93] as well as sternocleidomastoid and anterior scalene muscles [21]. The same phenomenon was observed in the upper trapezius during a 1 hour computer typing task maintaining a prolonged static posture [96] as well as during isometric contractions of the neck into extension and lateral flexion [97]'and during isometric circular contractions in the horizontal plane [73]. On the contrary, the deep cervical extensors, multifidus and semispinalis cervicis, were less activated during isometric extension performed in prone lying in patients with chronic neck pain compared to healthy controls, as demonstrated by O'Leary et al. [98]. In summary, a general pattern of increased activation of the superficial and decreased activation of the deep cervical muscles with a delayed onset and ofsett of muscle activity can be recognized in patients with neck pain.

1.5.4 Directional specificity of muscle activity

In healthy subjects, the ability to contract a muscle in well-defined preferred direction according to its anatomical position relative to the spine is a characteristic of all extensors [99, 100]. This so-called directional specificity increases in different neck muscles of healthy subjects with higher loads (e.g. 50 N versus 25 N) [100]. Splenius capitis is an exception with slightly variable preferred directions between different healthy subjects and with no increase in directional specificity at higher loads [100]. The directional specificity decreases with age in extension but not in flexion [101]. It is lower in patients with neck pain for example for the splenius capitis muscle and in sternocleidomastoid muscle compared to healthy controls [73, 92]. The lower directional specificity of the splenius capitis was positively correlated with the patients reported chronic neck pain and perceived disability and negatively correlated with the patients maximum cervical flexion force and even more with the total neck strength [73]. The sternocleidomastoid muscle, however, did not show similar correlations [73].

1.5.5 Coactivtion of muscles

The time simultaneous activation of agonist and antagonist muscles, called coactivation, is supposed to be a default strategy of the nervous system when confronted with uncertainty about the task, because learning of the motor task was accompanied by a reduction of coactivation and an increased use of reciprocal activation [102]. Coactivation of neck flexors and extensors in healthy subjects is less at high speed movements compared to middle and low speed suggesting feedback mechanisms as responsible for coactivation [103]. Increased coactivation is associated with pain and disability for example in splenius capitis and therefore an indicator for pathology [73]. Such a correlation however could not be found for sternocleidomastoid muscle probably because the reduction in neck flexion strength in the patient group was higher (31.7% less than controls) compared to extension (22.6% less than controls) and increased muscle coactivation seems to occur in the directions of leaststrength [73].

1.6 STRUCTURAL CHANGES IN THE NECK MUSCLES ASSOCIATED WITH PAIN

Fatty infiltration and changes in cross-sectional area (CSA) have been observed in the cervical muscles reflecting atrophy and degeneration. General fat infiltration in human skeletal muscle is variable for example between subjects of African origin, higher in women than men and largely influenced by genetic factors [104]. Muscle infiltration with fat tissue has been extensively described for the human supraspinatus in rotator cuff tears as an irreversible and usually progressive degenerative change ending in a definitive loss of muscular function [105]. Fat and fibrous tissue invade the space between the shortened muscle fibres as shown in infraspinatus tendon tears of the sheep (Fig. 1) [106].

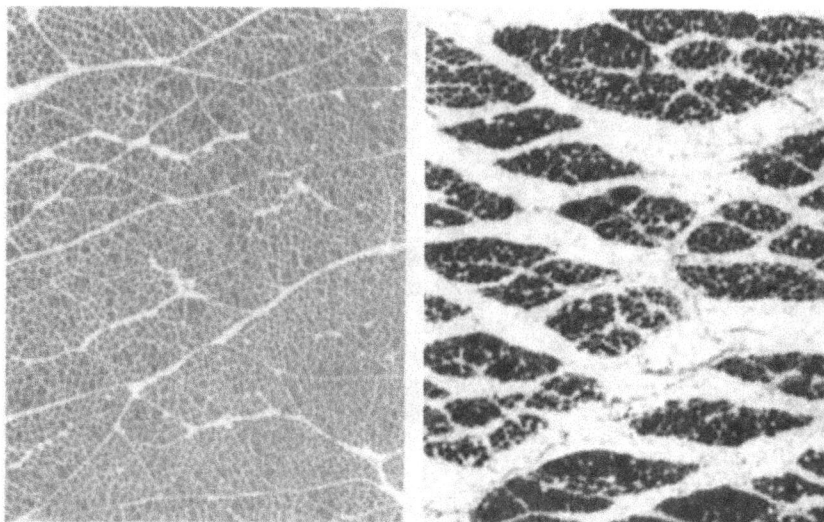

Fig. 1. Infraspinatus muscle of a sheep intact (left) and (right) after surgical tendon section left 40 weeks disconnected and then left 35 weeks after surgical repair reconnected. Note infiltration of fat (33 ± 8.7%) and connective tissue (12.9 ± 3.2%; together 45.9%) compared to 1.5 ± 0.5% and 2.4 ± 0.5% (together 3.9%) (From Meyer et al. 2004; with permission from the publisher)

In the human neck, the anterior muscles of patients with neck pain following a whiplash injury showed higher fat infiltration at the levels C2-3 and C5-6 compared to healthy controls, and more so in the deep longus capitis and longus colli than in the superficial sternocleidomastoid muscle [107]. In the cervical extensor muscles of patients with neck pain following a whiplash injury greater fat infiltration was observed compared to healthy controls, especially in the multifidus muscle between the levels C3 and C7 and in the semispinalis cervicis muscle mainly at the level of C3 (Fig. 2) [108]. In patients with insidious onset of neck pain, fat infiltration however has not been identified consistently [109]. Fat infiltration in the cervical extensor muscles was only weakly correlated to sensory, physical, kinaesthetic, and psychological features with cold pain threshold having the strongest correlation [110].

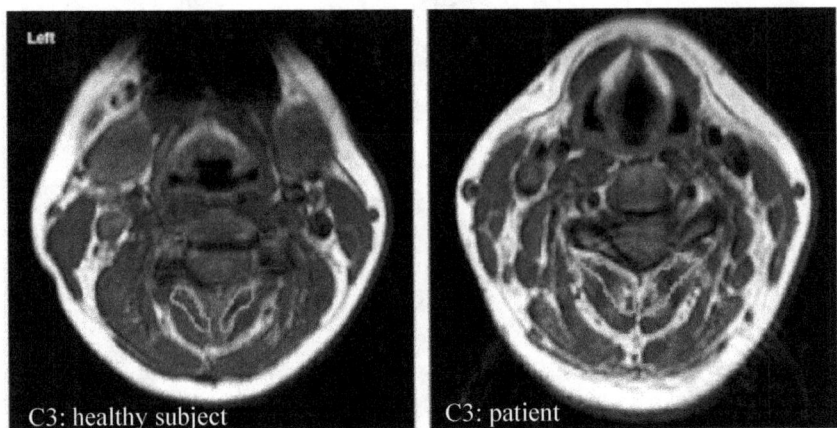

Fig. 2. Axial MRI scan at level C3 from a healthy subject and a patient
with neck pain after whiplash injury (WAD = whiplash associated
disorders). The line highlights the multifidus muscle. (from Elliott et al.
2006; with permission from the publisher)

It was suggested that fatty tissue infiltration of muscle in patients with chronic
neck pain following a whiplash injury may indicate non-recovery, but the
significance of this muscular degeneration is still unclear [110]. The association of
fatty infiltration with higher pain and disability and symptoms of post-traumatic
stress disorders suggests that such muscle changes may indicate poor functional
recovery [111]. This fatty infiltration especially in the deep cervical muscles might
partly explain the variable findings in cross-sectional area (CSA) measurements
(Fig. 3) found in the deep cervical extensors in patients with neck pain.

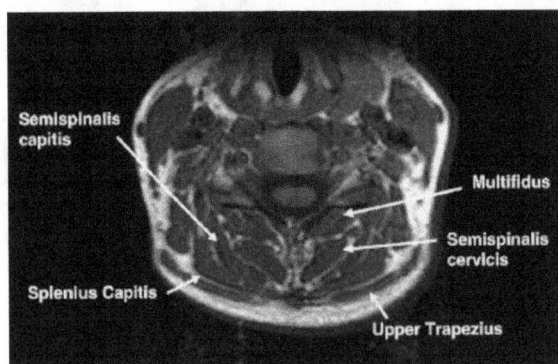

Fig. 3. T1-weighted axial MRI scan at the C6 segmental level in a healthy
control showing the cross-sectional areas of the cervical extensor muscles
(from Elliott et al. 2008; with permission from the publisher)

Semispinalis cervicis and multifidus together showed less CSA in patients with neck pain following a whiplash injury compared to healthy controls. The difference of about 6 mm^2 at level C2-3 and 2 mm^2 at level C5-6 showed a statistical significant difference [112]. It is close to the 2.2 mm^2 which are considered the minimum for real change when measuring muscle CSA of the semispinalis capitis muscle repeatedly with ultrasonography (Fig. 4) [113].

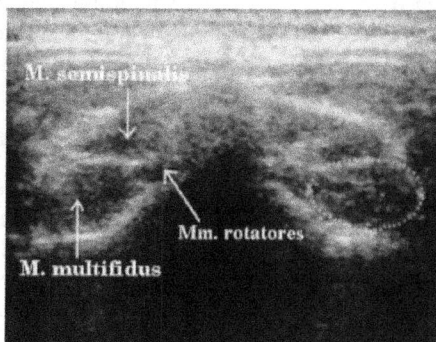

Fig. 4. Ultrasonogram of the cross-sectional area of the deep cervical extensors at level C4 in an asymptomatic subject (from Kristjansson 2004; with permission from the publisher)

Its clinical relevance therefore may be questioned [114]. The CSA of the multifidus muscle was also less in patients with neck pain following a whiplash injury [115] and patients with chronic non-traumatic neck pain [116] compared to healthy controls. Fighter pilots with chronic neck pain however showed even greater CSA of semispinalis cervicis and multifidus compared to asymptomatic fighter pilots [117]. Other neck extensors displayed lower or similar CSA in patients compared to healthy controls [61, 113, 118]. Asymptomatic women whose physical activity level in daily live was classified as low presented larger CSA of the cervical extensors compared to women with high activity levels [119]. Changes of CSA in the cervical extensors are consequently variable and non-conclusive regarding their significance for neck pain.

Evidence was found suggestive of transformation from fibre type I to type II (i.e. from slow to fast twitch fibres) in the cervical flexor and extensor muscles (suboccipital, splenius capitis, trapezius) of patients with neck pain, independent from the type of neck pathology [120]. In the 2-3 years following the onset of neck pain, a high amount of transitional type-IIC fibres could be found in the muscle which is a sign of on-going transformation of muscle fibres [120]. This reduction of tonic fibres might be reflected in the greater fatigue of the sternocleidomastoid and anterior scalene muscles in patients with neck pain [121]. The fiber distribution in many cervical muscles such as the semispinalis cervicis, however, has not been analyzed up to now [122]. Structural changes of the neck muscles in patients with neck pain such as fatty tissue infiltration of muscle tissue, altered CSA, and fibre type transformation, consequently, do not clearly explain the appearance or maintenance of neck pain.

1.7 SUMMARY OF MUSCLE CHANGES ASSOCIATED WITH NECK PAIN

Patients with neck pain show altered motor control of the cervical spine and a number of structural changes such as fatty infiltration, altered CSA, and fibre type transformation in the neck muscles. These structural alterations however are variable and do not clearly explain the patient's pain. Functional changes found in patients with neck pain include less strength and endurance, and altered activation strategies with mainly increased activity in the superficial muscles and decreased one in the deep muscles, lower directional specificity, and higher co-activation. These functional alterations may reflect changes in the pain modulating system including hypersensitivity [123] and offer many possibilities for clinical assessment and treatment of patients with neck pain [42]. Little however is known about the activation of the deep cervical extensors in patients with neck pain although anecdotally they are considered important for the rehabilitation of patients with neck pain [27]. This thesis therefore investigates a deep cervical extensor, the semispinalis cervicis, analyzing its neural control at different spinal levels in healthy subjects, its activation in patients with chronic neck pain compared to healthy controls and the influence of tissue tenderness as well as an exercise for the specific activation of semispinalis cervicis.

1.8 RATIONALE FOR THE FOCUS ON THE DEEP CERVICAL EXTENSORS

Much research has been performed to investigate changes in cervical flexor muscle control in patients with neck pain but only few studies have analyzed the extensors [42]. Those that have been performed have usually focused on the superficial extensors and typically show increased activity of the superficial cervical extensors compared to healthy controls [93, 96, 97]. The only study prior to this thesis on the deep cervical extensors in patients with chronic mechanical neck pain revealed that multifidus and semispinalis cervicis were less active compared to healthy controls. This was measured with T2 shift values pre-post an isometric extension of the neck in a neutral position in muscle functional Magnetic Resonance Imaging (mfMRI) [98]. Experimental pain provoked in the upper trapezius also reduced activity of the deep cervical extensors at level C7-T1 but not C2-3 in healthy subjects as measured by mfMRI [124]. The magnitude of T2 shift however required to justify clinical significance is still not known as stated by the authors [98]. Although this preliminary evidence suggests that the activity of the deep extensors may be lower in patients with neck pain, further research is necessary to better understand changes in the activation of the deep cervical extensors in patients with neck pain in order to be able to develop appropriate exercises. This thesis will contribute to this topic.

1.9 ANATOMY OF THE NECK EXTENSORS

The focus of this thesis is on the semispinalis cervicis. The relation of the semispinalis cervicis to the other cervical extensors will be described in the following. The posterior neck muscles, mainly extensors, are topographically organized in four muscle layers (Fig. 5) [99, 125]:

1. upper trapezius
2. splenius capitis and levator scapulae
3. semispinalis capitis
4. semispinalis cervicis, multifidus and rotatores

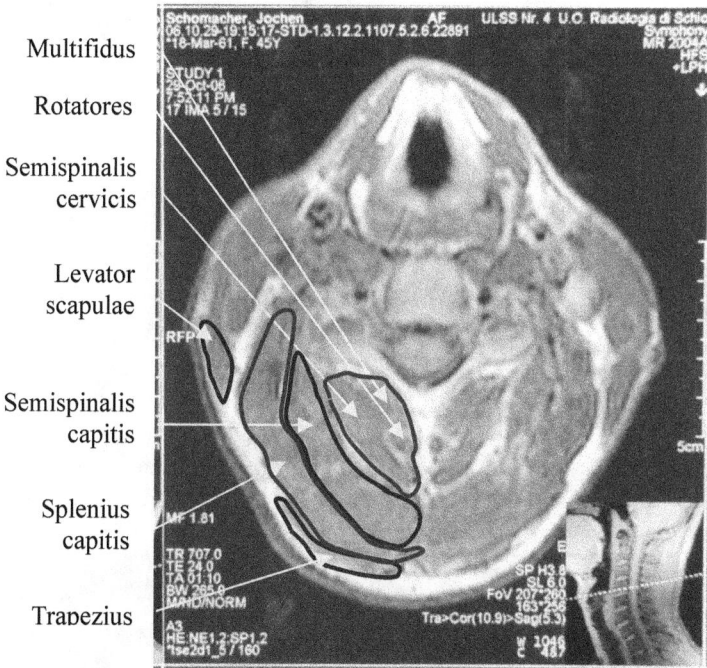

Fig. 5. MRI scan at the level C4 of a 45 year old healthy male subject showing the four layers of the extensor muscle group.

In the first layer, the upper trapezius (Fig. 6) acts mainly as a scapula stabilizer and only little on the head and neck with extension, ipsilateral sidebending and contralateral rotation [99, 126]. Some authors consider the trapezius an important muscle for head rotation due to its favourable moment arm for this movement [127].

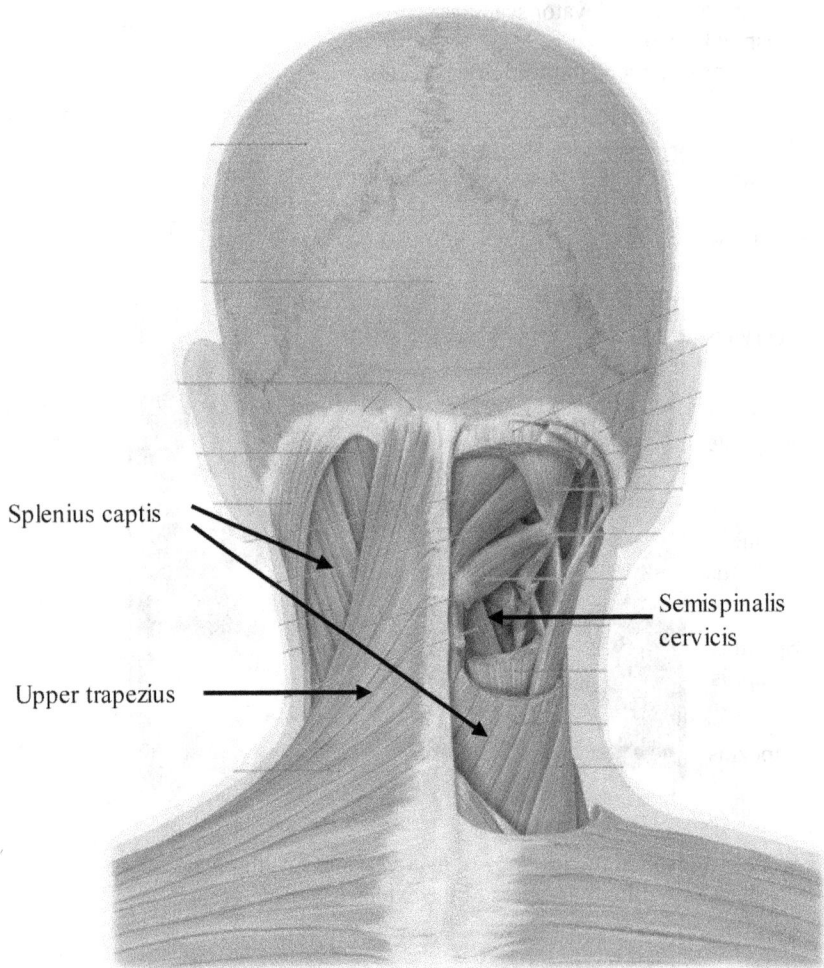

Fig. 6. Upper trapezius muscle in the superficial layer (left) and the deeper layers of the extensor muscles (right) (from: Schünke et al., 2005; with permission from the publisher)

Splenius capitis (Fig. 7) which will be investigated for comparison in the fourth study lies in the second layer. It is is active in extension, ipsilateral rotation and ipsilateral side bending, while some authors consider extension a secondary function [126]. Together with the other superficial extensors it is believed to be predominantly a prime mover due to large moment arms and attachments to the skull and trunk [100]. The more lateral lying levator scapulae in addition to its function on the scapula, extends, sidebends and rotates the cervical spine to the same side and might have a compressive action on the cervical spine [99, 126].

The third layer comprises the semispinalis capitis which extends sidebends and rotates the head to the opposite side, and in bilateral contraction it extends. Some authors consider it as part of the transversospinalis muscle system [128].

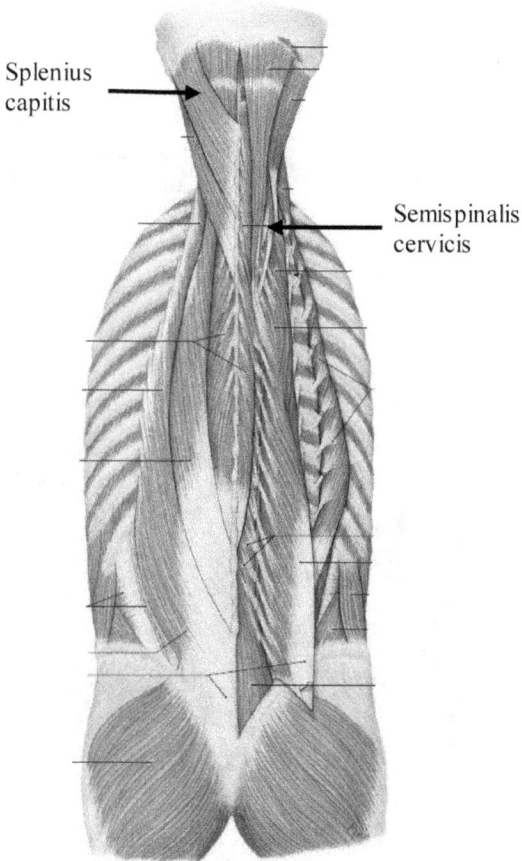

Fig. 7. Semispinalis cervicis and splenius capitis muscle in the context of the other posterior spinal muscles (from Tillmann, 2005; with permission from the publisher)

The fourth layer consists of the deep cervical extensors multifidus, rotatores and semispinalis cervicis (Fig. 8) [129, 130]. The rotatores are small and short muscles lying close to the vertebral arch and spinous process, medial to the multifidus. They rotate the vertebra to the opposite side. Multifidus is the deepest muscle close to the spine and has small moment arms [131]. Contrary to this muscle in the lumbar and thoracic region, the cervical multifidus originates directly from the capsules of the zygapophyseal joints which might explain its role in neck pain and injury [131]. The semispinalis cervicis which will be explored in all four studies of the thesis, forms together with the multifidus and rotatores the transversospinalis muscle which mainly extends the neck and participates in ipsilateral sidebending and contralateral rotation [99, 131].

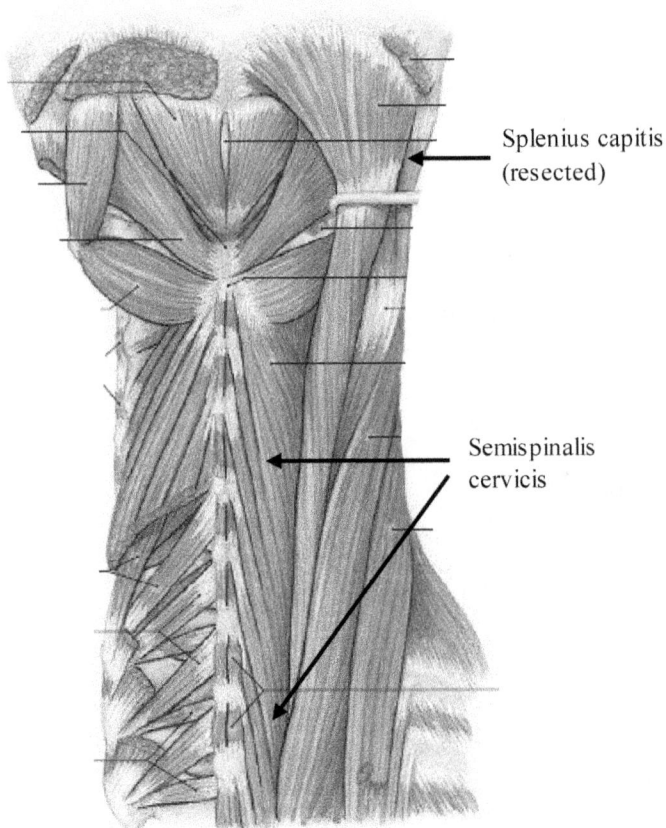

Splenius capitis (resected)

Semispinalis cervicis

Fig. 8. Semispinalis cervicis and splenius capitis muscle together with the other deep cervical extensors (from Tillmann, 2005; with permission from the publisher)

A topographical classification of the neck extensors respecting their function has also been proposed (Fig. 9) [42]. The extensors were divided into three muscle groups spanning

- the craniocervical region: suboccipital group

- the typical cervical region: semispinalis cervicis and multifidus with rotatores cervicis

- both regions: splenius capitis and cervicis, semispinalis capitis, and longissimus capitis (lying lateral)

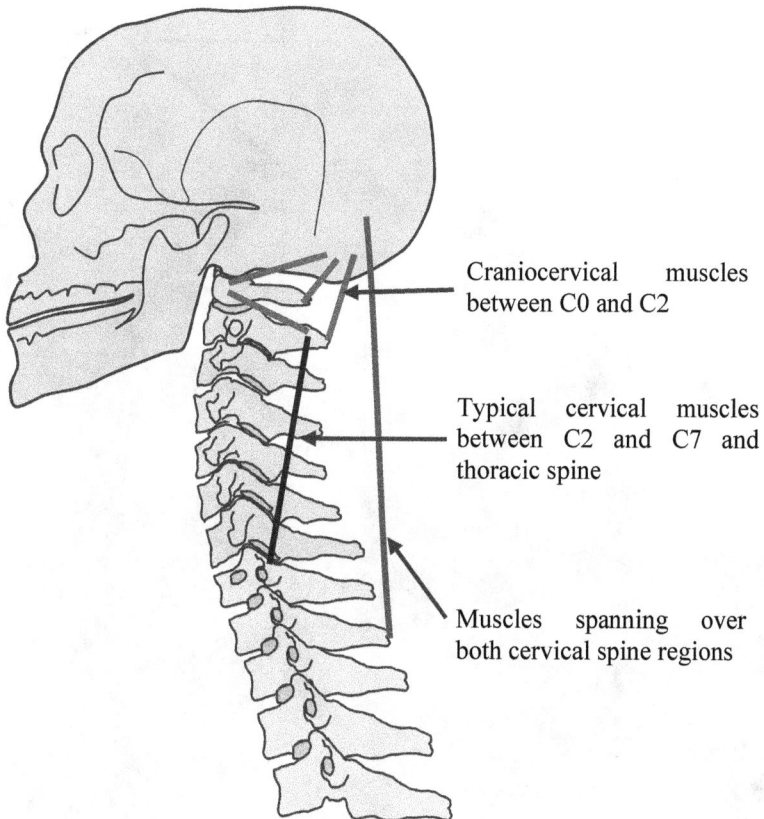

Craniocervical muscles between C0 and C2

Typical cervical muscles between C2 and C7 and thoracic spine

Muscles spanning over both cervical spine regions

Fig. 9. Classification of the neck extensors adapted from Jull et al. 2008

1.9.1 Semispinalis cervicis

The fibres of semispinalis cervicis (Fig. 10) have their origin at the transvers processes T1 to T5 or T6 and their insertion at the spinous processes of C2 to C5 [130] respectively to C7 [128, 132, 133] (Fig. 11). Their innervation comes from the medial branches of dorsal rami of the spinal nerves C3 to T6.

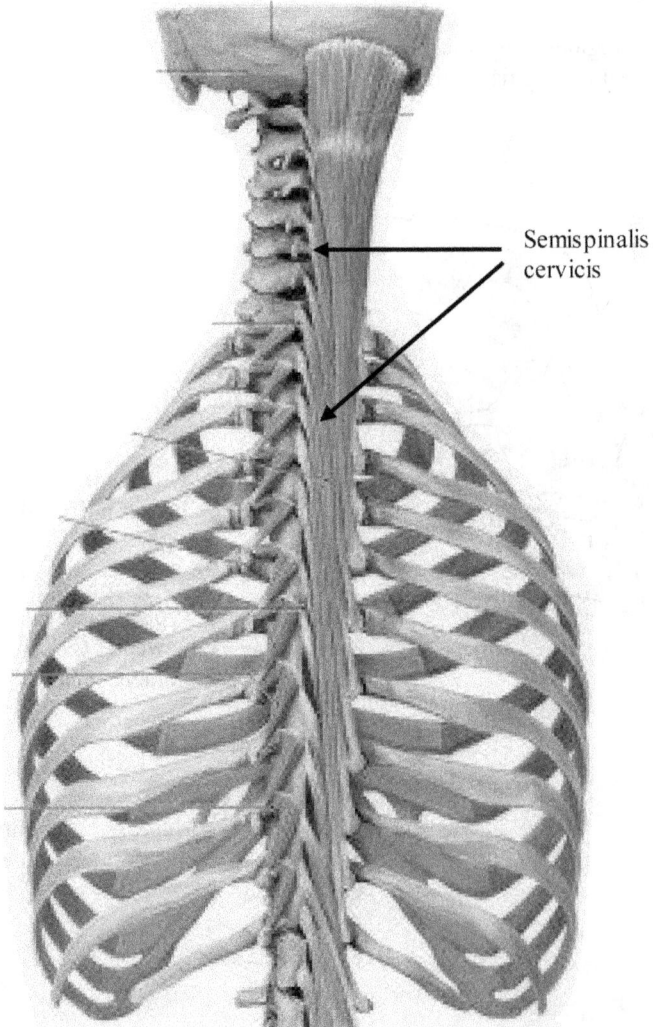

Fig. 10. Semispinalis cervicis muscle (from Schünke et al., 2005; with permission from the publisher)

A unilateral contraction of semispinalis cervicis produces extension with ipsilateral sidebending and contralateral rotation of the head while a bilateral contraction results in extension. Muscles with small moment arms and attachments to adjacent vertebrae are considered important stabilizers of the spine [134]. For the cervical extensors this applies to semispinalis cervicis together with the multifidus and semispinalis capitis muscles [100, 126]. The anatomy of semispinalis cervicis is similar to the one of multifidus [99, 131] which contains a high proportion (~70%) of slow twitch fibres [135]. The fibre composition of semispinalis cervicis is likely to be similar although no histological data on semispinalis cervicis has been reported.

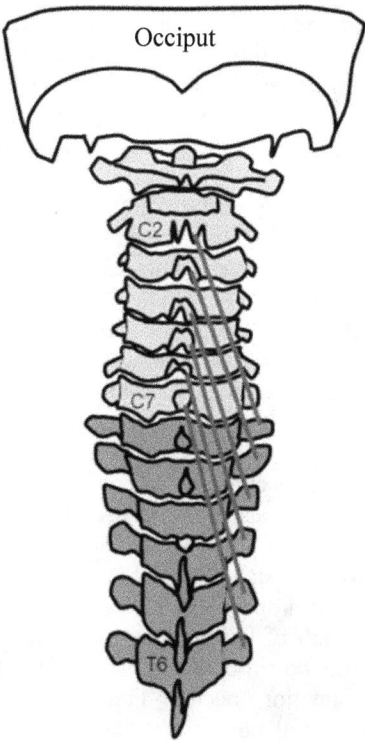

Fig. 11a. Schematic course of semi-spinalis cervicis muscle fascicles: dorsal view (based on Schünke 2000)

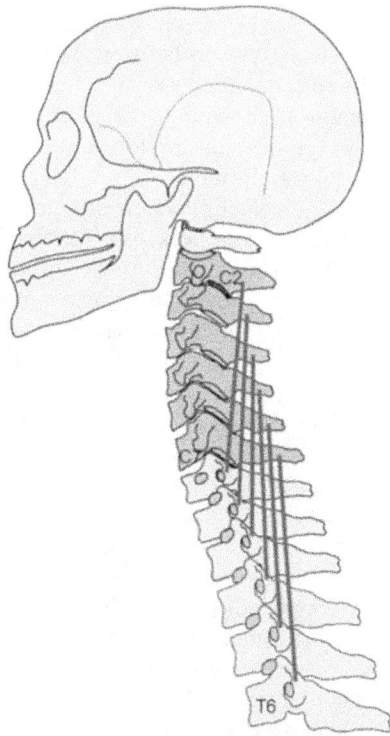

Fig. 11b. Schematic course of semi-spinalis cervicis muscle fascicles: lateral view (based on Schünke 2000)

In concert with the deep flexors longus capitis and longus colli, the semispinalis cervicis and multifidus form a muscular sleeve enclosing and stabilizing the cervical spine [99]. This is believed to prevent overloading of spinal structures with the risk of injury and pain [136]. MRI [137] and a model based analysis [127] have found semispinalis cervicis, splenius capitis, and semispinalis capitis to be the most effective extensors. The semispinalis cervicis was the first muscle to be activated during a static contraction into extension, followed by multifidus and semispinalis capitis and, finally, the trapezius, as measured with tissue velocity ultrasound imaging [138]. The multifidus was shown to be activated at level C4-C5 during right and left rotation probably to neutralize the flexion torque of prime rotators like sternocleidomastoid muscle [67].

In the thesis the semispinalis cervicis was selected for investigation of the deep cervical extensors because wire insertion was facilitated for several reasons:
1. The semispinalis cervicis is the first deep extensor muscle reached by a needle coming from the dorsal side of the neck. The risk of touching the dura mater with the insertion needle is consequently lower for the semispinalis cervicis than the multifidus.
2. The semispinalis cervicis muscle showed less fatty infiltration than multifidus in patients with neck pain following a whiplash injury compared to controls [108]. The risk of placing the tip of the wire into non contractile tissue was consequently lower for semispinalis cervicis than for multifidus.
3. The CSA of the semispinalis cervicis is larger than the one of multifidus [112, 119] and has a quite homogeneous distribution across spinal levels while most other extensor muscles including multifidus increased their CSA from the rostral to caudal direction in healthy women [119].

In study 4 the activation of the deep semispinalis cervicis was compared to the splenius capitis (Fig. 12). This superficial extensor muscle was chosen because it has a larger CSA than the upper trapezius (Elliott et al. 2007) and it acts on the head, while the upper trapezius acts more on the shoulder girdle [99, 126]. These advantages prevail the slightly variable directional specificity of splenius capitis [100]. Splenius capitis originates from the lower half of ligamentum nuchae and the spinous processes of C7 to T4. It attaches at the dorsal border of mastoid process and the lateral half or one-third of superior nuchal line below the sternocleidomastoid. Lateral branches of the dorsal rami of the middle cervical nerves innervate this muscle. Its unilateral contraction results in rotation and sidebending of the head and neck to the same side while a bilateral contraction provides extension [130].

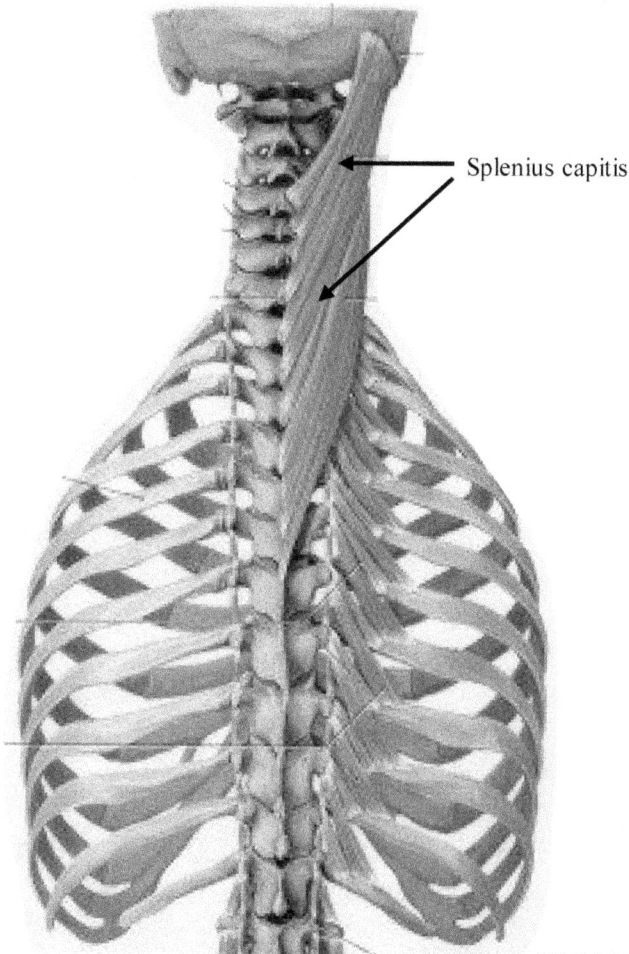

Fig. 12. Splenius capitis muscle (from: Schünke et al., 2005; with permission from the publisher)

In summary, the deep cervical extensors with semispinalis cervicis are important for stabilization and movement control of the cervical spine. The neural control of this muscle and the influence on neck pain on this control are the focus of this thesis.

Chapter 2.

Electromyographic assessment of the neural drive to muscle

Innovative non-invasive technology offers new possibilities for the analysis of muscle activation. The timing of muscle contraction for example can be examined with tissue velocity ultrasound imaging [138] and the muscle recruitment post exercise can be evaluated with muscle functional magnetic resonance imaging [139]. However, electromyography (EMG) still represents the best direct tool for analysis of muscle activation and was therefore selected as the main methodology in this thesis. The basic neurophysiology of muscle activation and EMG based outcomes of the studies will be explained in this chapter.

2.1 NEURAL DRIVE TO MOTOR UNITS

A motor unit (MU) is formed by one spinal motoneuron and all muscle fibres it innervates [140]. When a sufficiently high level of excitatory synaptic input is received by the motoneuron, it generates an action potential that causes its muscle fibres to contract. Higher synaptic input to one motoneuron results in an increase in the rate by which it generates action potentials, a phenomenon called rate coding or frequency coding. Higher synaptic input to the whole population of motoneurons results in activation of more motor units which is called recruitment. This summation in time (rate coding) and space (recruitment) of motor unit activation leads to muscle contractions for stabilization or movement of joints [141]. Muscle activation thus depends on the neural drive to the spinal motoneurons.

The motor cortex with its volitional control in collaboration with subcortical structures like basal ganglia sends its signals to the spinal motoneurons predominantly via monosynaptic projections [142, 143] but also via spinal interneurons organized in a premotoneural network [144] (Fig. 13.).

Motor cortex

Subcortical structures   Peripheral afferent feedback
(basal ganglia ...)   from extero- and proprioception

Spinal interneurons =
premotoneural network

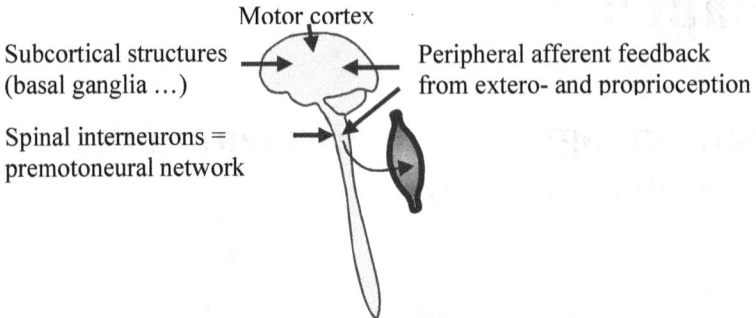

Fig. 13. Input to the spinal motoneuron

For example, the alpha-motoneurons of the first and second dorsal interosseous muscle of the hand [145] and the abductor digiti minimi [146] receive synaptic input directly from the motor cortex. In addition to this input from the brain, motoneurons also receive inhibitory and excitatory input from spinal interneurons and peripheral afferent feedback [147]. Afferents influencing the motoneurons of the cervical muscles for example come from the sense organs (exteroception) reflecting the orientation of the head and from the whole body (proprioception) reflecting the body's posture [148]. This is illustrated for example by the change in activity of the cervical erector spinae [149] and the deep cervical flexor muscles in different sitting positions [150].

Muscle activity can be studied at several levels, including the level of mechanical output (force, movement) and the myoelectrical activity using EMG. Furthermore, from intramuscular EMG (iEMG) recordings the activity of single motor units can be identified. This provides the most direct measure of the neural drive to the muscle [151] and is used to study for example the effects of disease (of muscle or neuron) [152], fatigue and aging [153]. In addition, the analysis of the neural drive to muscles allows the construction of conceptual models of motor unit control strategies [154]. This was applied in study 1 of this thesis.

2.2 ELECTROMYOGRAPHY

Electromyography (EMG) is the recording of action potentials (AP) of muscle fibres that are firing individually or in groups near the electrode [155]. The electrode can be inserted into the muscle via a needle (needle EMG or iEMG) or pasted on the skin (surface EMG = sEMG). In non-pathologic conditions the AP of the muscle fibres is a response to the AP of its innervating motoneuron [155]. The resting muscle normally shows no APs, i.e. no EMG activity [155]. The variable space between the active neuron and the receptive electrode allows several factors to influence the recorded electrical signal like the conductibility of the tissue between the muscle fibre and the electrode, the distribution of the motor unit territories, and the recruitment of new motor units over time as a consequence of fatigue [156]. In addition, the distance between the electrode and the AP of the muscle fibre as well as the muscle fibre size determine the amplitude of the AP [152, 157]. The higher this distance for example the lower the amplitude and the rate of rise of the positive-negative inflection of the externally recorded AP [155]. Further, the bigger the muscle fibre the higher the AP amplitude [153, 155]. The amplitude of interference EMG therefore does not reflect directly the strength of a muscle. Size and shape of the potential normally remain constant over the firing time [155], but changes can occur [158].

The interference pattern of EMG describes the superposition of action potentials from different motor units [152]. The amplitude of a spike in the EMG interference pattern might consequently be composed by superposition of several single action potentials. Increasing the number of activated motor units and their firing rate (spatial and temporal recruitment) however will not only increase the amplitude of the EMG interference pattern, but also the contraction strength of the muscle. The interference pattern is not suited for the analysis of individual MUAP [159] although specific methods like the Convolution Kernel Compensation method allow identification of the discharge pattern of single motor units from high-density sEMG [160]. Investigation of single action potentials is generally done by iEMG. Under normal circumstances, single muscle fibre action potentials (MFAPs) are too small to be detected, but all the muscle fibres of a motor unit discharge in near synchrony, so that their sum results in a single action potential, the motor unit action potential (MUAP) [155]. A MUAP therefore is the summation of the MFAPs of the fibres being near the recording electrode (primarily those within 0.5 mm) and consequently not of all fibres belonging to one motor unit [153]. Individual MUAPs can be best observed when a muscle contracts minimally [155]. At higher efforts more MUs are activated and interfere with each other.

2.2.1 Analysis of single MUAPs

Stimulation of a single neuron produces an action potential which reflects the change in the electric membrane potential. A sequence of APs generated by a neuron forms a so-called spike-train, called for the motoneuron the motor unit action potential train (MUAPT) [141]. These spike trains are the basis for neural coding and information transfer in the nervous system. Spike trains can form different patterns like rhythmic spiking and bursting, and are often considered an oscillatory activity[161]. Different types of information about the neural drive to the muscle can be derived from the spike trains. It must be remembered however, that the EMG wire detects only a few action potentials which are not necessarily representative for all fibres in the motor unit and not for all motor units in the muscle [154]. The parameters deduced from the spike trains in this thesis are explained in the following.

2.2.2 Discharge rate

The discharge or firing rate of motor units is defined as the number of neuronal signals (action potentials) generated per second from a neuron and expressed in frequency measured in Hertz (Hz) [155] or pulses per second (pps) [142]. MUAPs of normal voluntary activity show a semi rhythmic pattern and a relatively constant frequency [155]. The initial firing rate of a motor unit, i.e. the frequency of firing when a motor unit starts to be recruited (= begins to discharge) [153] is usually between 5 to 8 pps [152, 155]. During mild contractions in normal limb muscles the discharge rate is usually between 7-10 Hz and goes up to 16 Hz for motor units in cranial muscles [152, 155, 162]. As the magnitude of the synaptic input to the motorneuron increases, the firing rate of individual motor units increases up to 20 – 40 Hz. The maximum discharge rate of motor units is in average about 20 – 30 Hz for sustained efforts at 80-100% of maximum activation of the muscle [102, 155] while motor units in brief high-level contractions can achieve 65-100 Hz [102].

The characteristics of the discharge rate of a motor unit can be studied by generating histograms of the times between each action potential, the so-called interspike intervals (ISI). The result is an interspike-interval histogram [141, 163, 164] (Fig. 14).

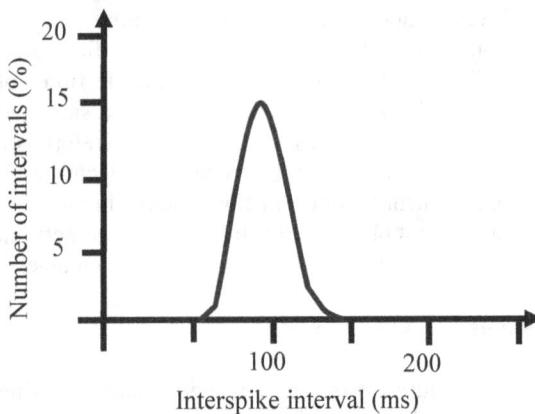

Fig. 14. Schematic interspike interval histogram

The variability of the discharge rate during sustained contractions can be measured by the variability of ISI [165]. It is computed by dividing the standard deviation of ISI through the mean of ISI (ISI variability = ratio (%) between SD and mean of ISI).This coefficient of variation of ISI is a measure of relative discharge rate variability and has an effect on the force fluctuations during steady contractions [165]. The coefficient of variation of ISI is reflected in the width of the peak in the ISI-histogram in the sense that a narrow peak represents a small variability and vice versa.

2.2.3 Recruitment of motor units

Motor units are recruited according to Henneman's size principle [166, 167]. First small units with a low recruitment threshold are activated. They innervate slow-twitch muscle fibres which provide low force but high endurance. At higher levels of synaptic input to the motor units larger units are recruited. They innervate fast-twitch muscle fibres which develop higher force but exhibit less endurance [162].

The level of force generated by the muscle, at which a motor unit starts to be recruited is referred to as its recruitment threshold (Fig. 15). This point can be expressed in Newton or in % of the maximal voluntary contraction (= MVC) [168].

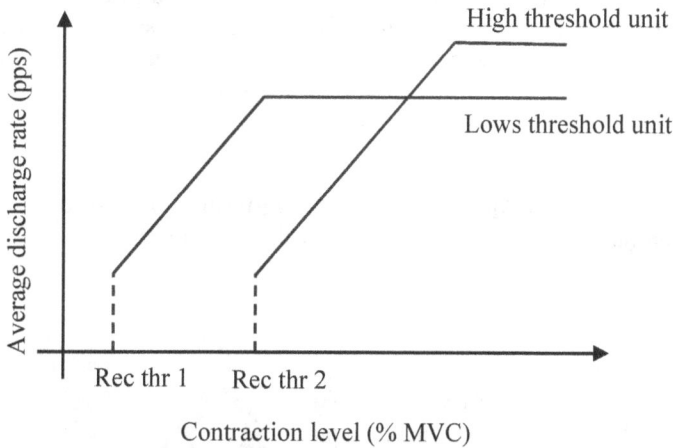

Fig. 15. Schematic representation of two motor units with their respective recruitment thresholds (Rec. thr.).

2.2.4 Analysis of motor unit population input

Numerous motor units fire consistently during sustained force contractions [169]. Normally motor units fire randomly in order to produce a smooth motor output which is supported by the filtering performed by the compliant and viscous muscle components [169]. Common input to a motor neuron pool is reflected in the discharge pattern as an increased tendency for synchronized firing of the motoneurons [169, 170]. Motor unit synchronization consequently is the tendency of two motor units to fire dependently from each other more often than it would happen by chance [169, 171].

The degree of motor unit synchronization during sustained contractions can be analyzed with cross-correlation histograms of single motor unit spike trains [157, 159, 170]. It measures the similarity of two waveforms as a function of a time-lag applied to one of them . When two spike trains are independent from each other, the cross-correlation histogram between those spikes trains will be flat, that is the cross-correlation function is a constant. When the cross-correlation is not flat, some functional correlation can be assumed between the analysed two motor units.

The cross-correlation analysis estimates the strength of the common input to two motor neurons [171]. This synchronization can be quantified by the Common Input Strength index (CIS) [172] which denotes the number of synchronous discharges in excess of chance per second. In the cross-correlation histogram the sharp peak has often a width of less than ± 6 ms which denotes short-term synchronization [169]. Short-term synchronization indicates an input to the motor units through branches from a single presynaptic neuron [171]. In the relatively rare broad-peak synchronization the amplitude peaks are lower, with similar width and centred at latencies ranging from 8 to 76 ms [169]. Broad-peak synchronization indicates an input to the motor units from interneurons that are themselves activated by single presynaptic neurons (Fig. 16) [171]. The functional role of motor unit synchronization is not fully known [102] but has been suggested to be to increase the strength or to promote skilled muscle synergies [171].

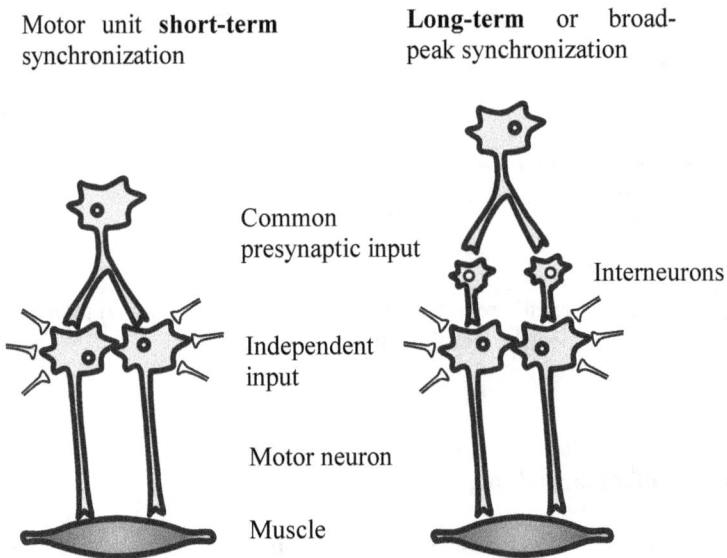

Motor unit **short-term** synchronization

Long-term or broad-peak synchronization

Common presynaptic input

Interneurons

Independent input

Motor neuron

Muscle

Fig. 16. Neurological pathways for short-term and broad-peak synchronization (adapted from Semmler 2002)

The tendency for MUs to display similar slow modulations of their discharge rates (= common fluctuations/oscillations in the mean firing rate) is referred to as the common drive [142]. Similarly to motor unit synchronization it relies on the cross correlation function, but instead of using the motor unit spike trains, smoothed discharge rates are used [169]. The oscillations characterized by the common drive have been suggested to be a reflection of the conscious, compensatory changes in the descending cortical drive to the muscles, when for example maintaining a constant isometric force.

Synchronization was evaluated for pairs of units within the individual recording site and for pairs across recording sites. The quality of estimate of the strength of motor unit synchronization from motor units recorded in one single site strongly depends on the accuracy of the decomposition program. The applied decomposition software has been shown to be highly accurate, so that estimates of synchronization from a single electrode site are appropriate [159](Dideriksen et al. 2009), as recently discussed [173]. The degree of motor unit synchronization was estimated by generating cross-histograms (±50 ms relative to the reference motor unit discharge; bin width: 1 ms) of all combinations of motor unit pairs [142, 172]. Cross-histograms with an average bin-count of less than 4 were excluded from the analysis [142]. The width of the synchronous peak in the cross-histogram was identified using the cumulative sum [174]. Synchronization was quantified by the Common Input Strength (CIS) index [172], which denotes the number of synchronous discharges in excess of chance per second. A significant synchronous peak in the cumulative sum function was defined as an increase of at least three standard deviations above the mean of the first 30 bins [175].

While the cross-correlation analysis estimates the temporal similarity of the output of two motor neurons, coherence analysis describes the frequencies of common input to two motor units by describing the similarity of two motor unit spike trains across the spectral frequencies of the signal (Fig. 17).

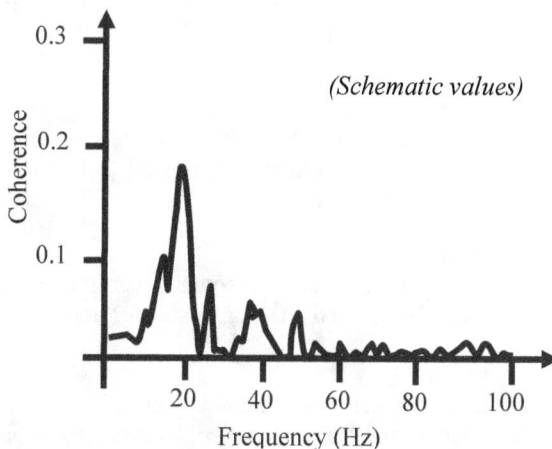

Fig. 17. Schematic representation of a coherence analysis

Therefore, coherence analysis provides additional information about the synaptic inputs responsible for motor unit synchronization that cannot be obtained solely from cross-correlation analysis [176]. Coherence between motor unit pairs implies some common periodicity of presynaptic input [171]. For example, a significant coherence at frequencies of 1–12 Hz and 16–32 Hz during voluntary isometric abduction of the index finger has been observed [171]. Frequencies between 16 and 32 Hz belong to the so-called Beta-band which in EEG analysis is believed to be of high functional significance in the generation of voluntary movement [177] meaning that a significant coherence between two spike trains indicates a functional relevant common descending input to the two motor neurons. The coherence was estimated as the ratio of the squared magnitude of the cross-spectra of two spike trains and the product of their autospectra [178]. The peak value of coherence in the band 16-32 Hz was used to quantify the strength of common input in the beta band.

2.3 AIMS AND OUTLINE OF THIS THESIS

The general aim of this thesis is to investigate the activation of the semispinalis cervicis muscle. Four experiments were conducted to investigate the neural control of this muscle and potential changes in control in patients with neck pain. Further a final study was undertaken to assess whether selective exercise could be used to accentuate the activation of the semispinalis cervicis muscle (Fig. 18). The specific aims of each study are described in the following.

Study 1
Is there an independent neural drive to different fascicles of semispinalis cervicis?

Study 2
Is the activity of semispinalis cervicis lower in patients with neck pain compared to asymptomatic individuals at level C3?

Study 3
Is the activity of semispinalis cervicis related to pressure pain sensitivity at levels C2 and C5?

Study 4
Can the deep semispinalis cervicis be activated relative to the superficial splenius capitis in patients with neck pain?

Fig. 18. Outline of the thesis

Study 1: Recruitment of motor units in two fascicles of the semispinalis cervicis muscle

The semispinalis cervicis is built up of different fascicles spanning over different spinal segments. This raises the question whether the innervation of the fascicles is influenced by the mechanical requirements which are different in the middle and lower cervical spine. The behaviour of single motor units of semispinalis cervicis at two spinal levels was consequently investigated in healthy subjects. It was hypothesized that there is an independent neural drive to different fascicles of the muscle according to their mechanical needs and advantages.

Study 2: Chronic trauma-induced neck pain impairs the neural control of the deep semispinalis cervicis muscle

The directional specificity and mean activity of the semispinalis cervicis muscle was assessed in patients with neck pain and healthy controls as they performed multidirectional isometric contractions of their neck muscles. It was hypothesized that activity and directional specificity were less in patients with neck pain compared to healthy controls.

Study 3: Localized pain sensitivity is associated with reduced activation of the semispinalis cervicis muscle in patients with neck pain

Various factors including sensitization of the nervous system might influence muscle activity and partially explain the variability in activation of the semispinalis cervicis in patients with neck pain. Pain sensitivity can be assessed by the pressure pain threshold. In this study PPT were measured over the zygapophyseal joints at the levels C2 and C5. EMG amplitude and directional specificity of semispinalis cervicis were measured at the same spinal levels. It was hypothesized that the pressure pain thresholds were lower in patients and positively related to the EMG activity and directional specificity of semispinalis cervicis at both spinal levels.

Study 4: Localised resistance selectively activates the semispinalis cervicis muscle in patients with neck pain

In studies 2 and 3 it was shown that the activation of the semispinalis cervicis is lower in patients with neck pain compared to healthy controls. This study investigated whether an exercise with manual resistance applied to the neck or head could be used to selectively activate the semispinalis cervicis muscle relative to the more superficial extensor, the splenius capitis in patients with neck pain. It was hypothesized that a manual resistance at the vertebral arch would increase the activation of semispinalis cervicis compared to general resistance at the head.

Chapter 3.

Methodology

The methods of the four studies of this thesis are described in the following. Appendix 1 provides a brief overview.

3.1 SUBJECTS

Women suffer from neck pain more frequently than men [28] and were investigated in this thesis. The pathophysiological mechanisms of musculoskeletal disturbances in chronic neck pain syndromes are independent of the aetiology [179]. Some studies report no difference between patients with chronic neck pain of insidious onset or whiplash associated disorders regarding range of motion, peak velocity, smoothness of movement, and head repositioning acuity [180]. Changes in motor control strategies following neck pain of insidious or traumatic onset are not necessarily related to a history of neck trauma or current pain intensity, but more likely due to the long duration of pain [123]. Therefore, the results of this thesis which are mainly related to neck pain of traumatic origin are probably transferable to patients with non-traumatic neck pain.

Patients were recruited from a pain clinic and through advertisement in newspapers. Control subjects were recruited via advertising at Aalborg University. The inclusion criteria for the patients were age between 18 and 45 years, duration of pain over 3 months and a pain intensity of equal or more than 2.5 on a visual analogue scale. The healthy subjects of the same range of age had not to have any neck pain and no history of neck surgery or neurological disorders. Exclusion criteria for all participants were any complaints of neurological signs and/or neurological signs and/or a history of cervical spine surgery. Due to the invasive nature of the experiments the number of participants was limited for ethical reasons. Fifteen healthy volunteers were recruited in study 1 (7 women), 20 women in study 2 (10 patients), 19 women in study 3 (10 patients) and 10 female patients in study 4. Patients of study 4 were the same as in study 2 as both studies were performed simultaneously. Five patients of study 2 also volunteered for study 3 and were accepted due to recruitment difficulties. All participants had to be able to accomplish the test movements. Furthermore, each participant had to be able to understand the oral and written information on the experiment and to sign the informed consent form.

3.2 ULTRASOUND GUIDED INTRAMUSCULAR EMG (STUDIES 1-4)

Needle insertion into the semispinalis cervicis and splenius capitis muscles in this project followed standard procedures for iEMG [155]. Wire electrodes made of Teflon-coated stainless steel (diameter: 0.1 mm; A-M Systems, Carlsborg, WA) were inserted via a 27-gauge hypodermic needle. In this thesis ultrasonography was used to guide needle insertion for exact wire placement according to the literature [67, 100, 181]. Guidance of needle insertion by ultrasonography is an alternative to computerized tomography, which is costly and associated with ionization of the patient [99]. The gold standard for visualization of the cervical muscles is MRI which however is much more expensive than ultrasonography and does not allow guidance of needle insertion [115, 182, 183]. Ultrasonography applies ultrasound waves on the body and builds from its reflexions an image [184]. The fascia layers separating the extensor muscles produce an echo, i.e. they are echogenic. They reflect the ultrasound wave more than muscles and appear whiter than muscles in the ultrasound image (Fig. 19) [125, 184].

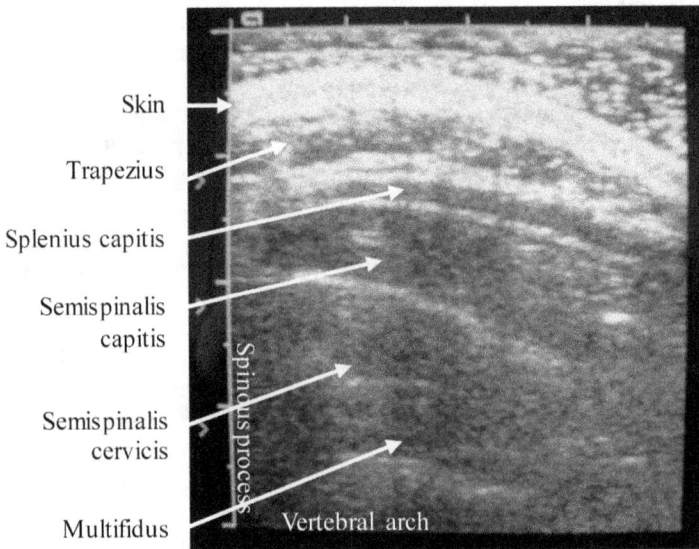

Fig. 19. Ultrasonography cross-section of the right side of a 22 year old healthy female at level C5 without squeezing the tissues.

Ultrasonography is a valid and reliable method for measuring muscle thickness and CSA of the deep cervical extensors [115] and other neck muscles – for review see Javanshir [183]. CSA measurement of the deep flexor longus colli however is questionable [185]. It is important to apply a constant pressure to the transducer because a strong pressure can flatten for example the human deltoid muscle up to 50% (Fig. 20) [186]. Identification of the insertion needle is difficult on a static image, but becomes easier while moving the needle.

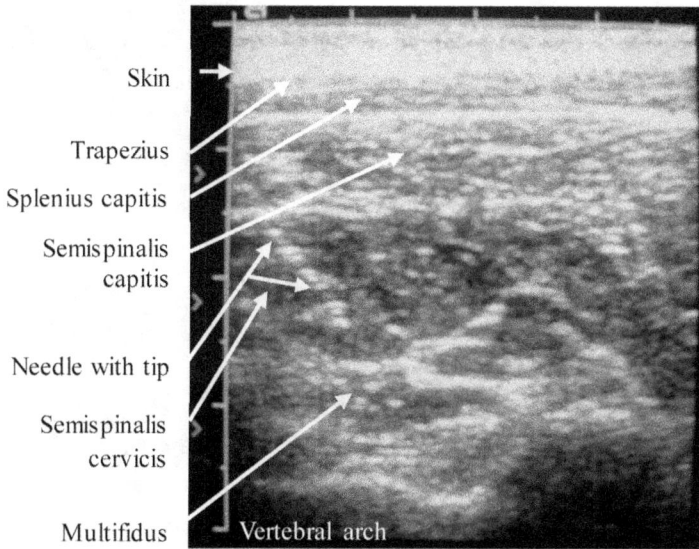

Fig. 20. Ultrasonography cross-section of the right side of a 28 year old healthy man at level C5 with squeezing the tissues. Note the flat shape on top of the picture compared to figure 19.

According to guidelines elaborated on CT scans of the neck and on human cadavers the puncture point for semispinalis cervicis lies 1.5 cm lateral to the median line and the puncture angle is 90° to the frontal plane [187, 188]. For splenius capitis a puncture point close to the previous one and an oblique puncture angle of approximately 45° analogous to the one for semispinalis capitis [187] were chosen because no guidelines could be found for this muscle. After approximate insertion of the carrier needle the correct position was guided by ultrasonography.

The fascia between the three deep neck extensors semispinalis cervicis, multifidus and rotatores is often difficult to distinguish with ultrasonography [115, 125]. The fascia however between the semispinalis capitis and semispinalis cervicis contains blood vessels [187] and is always clearly visible. The biggest vessel is the deep cervical artery (arteria cervicalis profunda) which supplies the deep cervical extensor muscles (Fig. 21) [189]. Visualization of this artery with Doppler sonography during the ultrasound scanning helped for identification of semispinalis cervicis muscle which lies ventrally to the fascia that contains the artery.

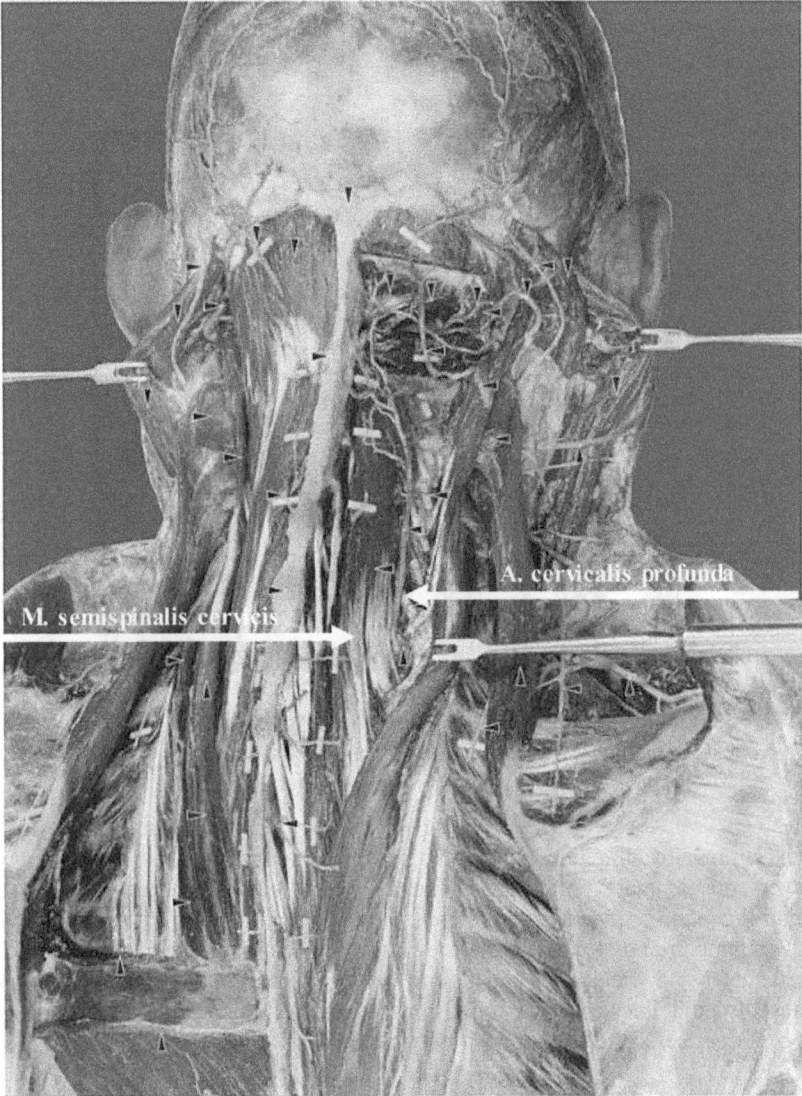

Fig. 21. Arteria cervicalis profunda
(from Thiel 2003; with permission from the publisher)

The deep cerival artery arises generally from the costocervical trunk and runs up in the fascia between the semispinalis capitis and semispinalis cervicis at the levels C7 to C2 (Fig. 22-23 [190].

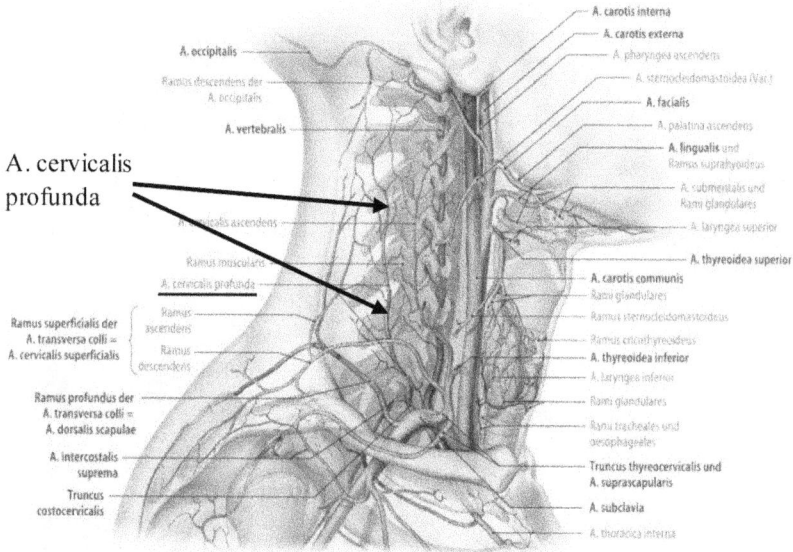

Fig. 22. Arteria cervicalis profunda (from Tillmann 2005; with permission from the publisher)

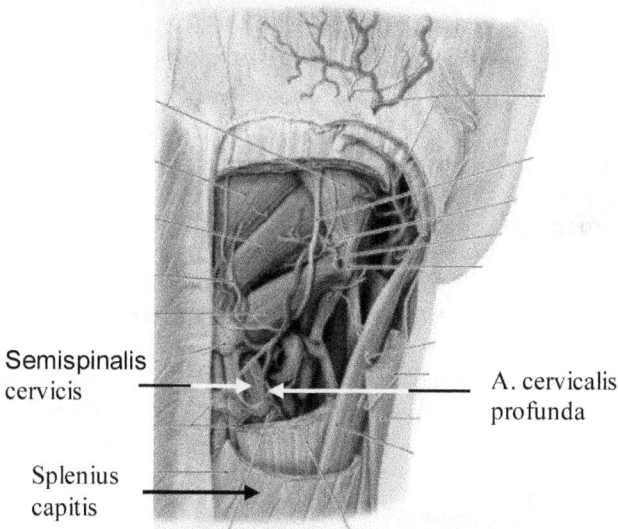

Fig. 23. Arteria cervicalis profunda between semispinalis capitis and semispinalis cervicis muscle (from Schünke et al. 2005; with permission from the publisher).

In order not to puncture the deep cervical artery it was visualized with Doppler sonography during the ultrasound scanning (Fig. 24). Insertion of the carrier needle was performed medial to the artery with a distance of more than 1 cm. The risk of hitting the blood vessels causing a painful haematoma was regarded as very unlikely in a cadaver study [187, 188].

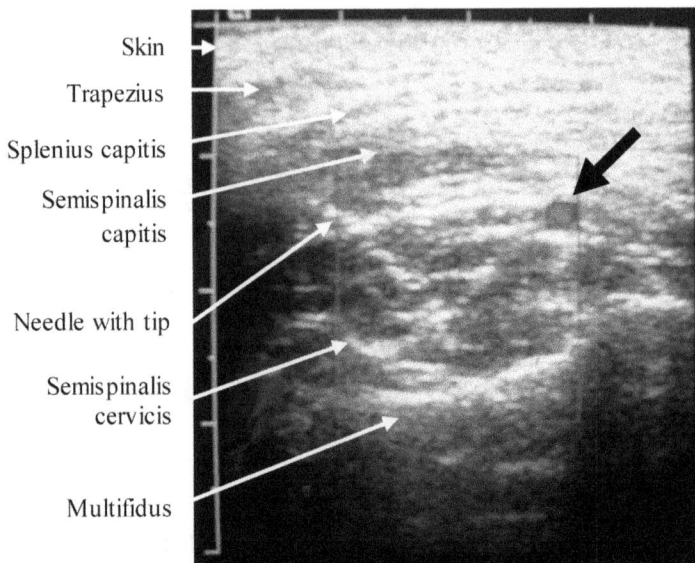

Fig. 24. Horizontal section at level C5 in a 23 year old healthy male with the arteria cervicalis profunda (= dot with arrow) and the needle in the semispinalis cervicis muscle.

The most cranial insertion of semispinalis cervicis is at the spinous process of C2 [132] where the deep extensors can be surrounded by fat tissue (Fig. 25). Identification of semispinalis cervicis at this level consequently is difficult [108, 191]. The spinous process level used in the current project however is slightly below the vertebral body level used in the MRI studies cited above. In case semispinalis cervicis was not clearly detectable at level C2, the ultrasound transducer was moved caudally until the muscle was clearly visible and wire insertion was made at this point.

In order to detect action potentials of individual motor units in the first study, the end of the wire was cut to expose only the cross section. For obtaining interference EMG in the other experiments, the insulation was removed from the end of the wire for approximately 3-4 mm.

Wires were inserted on the the side of greatest pain for the patients since in the lumbar spine the atrophy of multifidus muscle was confined predominantly to one level in the symptomatic segment on the side ipsilateral to the symptoms [192, 193]. It was hypothesized that it might be similar in the cervical spine although no corresponding studies were found. Healthy subjects were measured on the right side since the CSA of the multifidus, semispinalis cervicis and semispinalis capitis muscles was greater on the right side in healthy women [119]. The levels of C2, C3 and C5 were selected as the sites for needle insertion (Fig. 25).

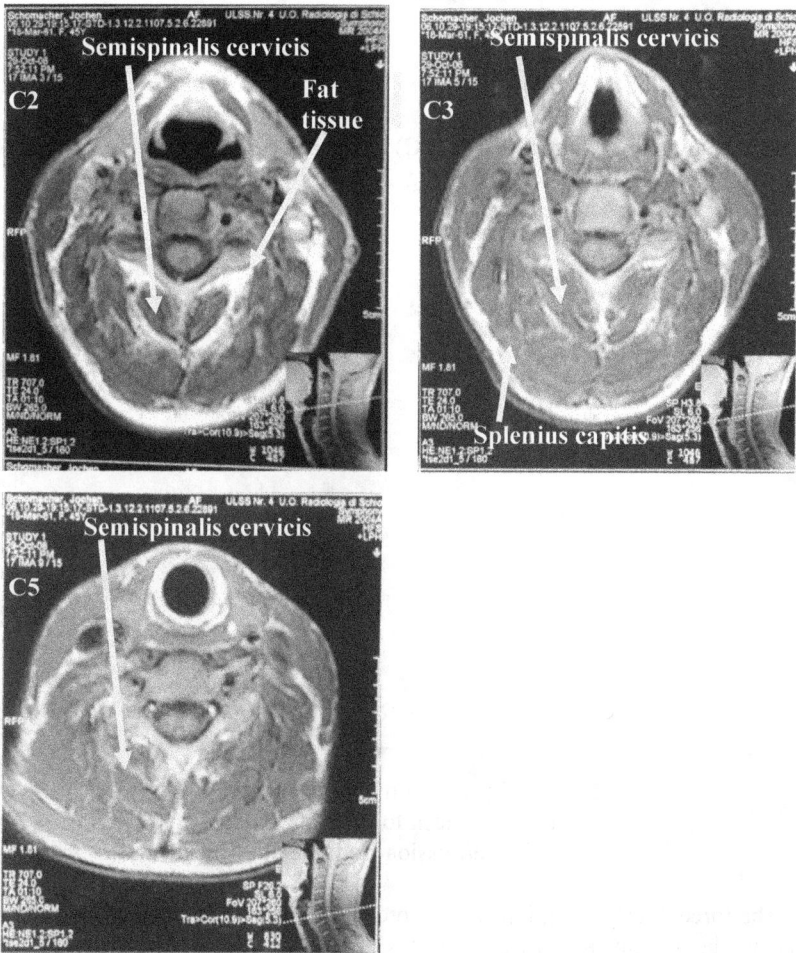

Fig. 25. MRI horizontal sections of the neck in a 45 year old healthy man with the muscles at spinal levels C2, C3, and C5 investigated in this thesis.

Using medial branch blocks of the zygapophyseal joints the levels C2-C3 and C5-C6 have shown to be the most frequently painful segments below C2 in patients with neck pain [47, 48, 194]. Also in a clinical examination C2-3 was the most symptomatic segment in a group of patients with chronic neck pain [25]. One reason for frequent pain in the lower cervical spine segments might be that the physiological limits of extension are often exceeded at these levels during whiplash trauma [52] causing facet joint injuries most frequently in C5-C6 and C6-C7 segments [55]. Furthermore, structural changes such as lower cross-sectional area (CSA) of semispinalis cervicis were found in patients with neck pain following a whiplash injury compared to healthy controls at the vertebral levels C3, C5 and C6 but not at levels C4 and C7, which might reflect segment specific muscle wasting [112]. For these reasons, levels C2, C3, and C5 were selected for investigation.

3.3 FORCE (STUDIES 1-3)

Maximum voluntary contractions (MVC) of the neck extensors were performed in a multidirectional neck force device (Fig. 26) (Aalborg University, Denmark) [92].

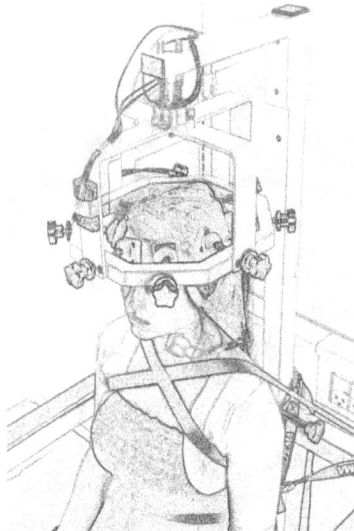

Fig. 26. Device for the measurement of multidirectional neck force (from Falla et al., 2010; with permission from the publisher)

The force device is equipped with force transducers (strain gauges) to measure force in the sagittal and coronal planes. The electrical signals from the strain gauges were amplified (OT Bioelettronica, Torino, Italy) and their output was displayed on an oscilloscope as visual feedback to the subject. Following a period of familiarization with the measuring device and a period to practice the desired contractions, subjects performed neck extensions at maximum force separated by 1 min of rest. Verbal encouragement was provided to the subject. The highest value of force recorded over repeated efforts of the maximum contractions of 5 s each was selected as the maximal force. Three MVCs were tested in the healthy subjects of study 1 without the inserted EMG wires because EMG signals were not normalized. In study 2 subjects were asked for only 2 MVCs as the variability of repeated MVC measurements was seen not to be high and in order to avoid unnecessary pain provocation in the participating patients. In this study MVC was tested with the inserted wires in order to allow normalization of the subsequently recorded EMG signals. In study 3 and 4 no MVC was tested as the absolute data have been used. In order to be able to compare the EMG amplitude at a percentage of MVC between subjects in the second experiment of study 1, the ARV computed at these force levels was normalized with respect to the ARV obtained during the MVC, that is the submaximal effort value was divided by the maximal effort value (for example 30% MVC divided by 100% MVC) and this ratio was compared between patients and controls.

3.4 PRESSURE PAIN THRESHOLD (PPT) (STUDY 3)

The point at which a person starts to feel pressure as painful is called the pressure pain threshold [195] and is measured with an algometer. This is a pressure-sensitive strain gauge situated at the end of a bar which is connected to an amplifier indicating the pressure in kPa [195]. In this project, an electronic algometer, with a probe surface of $1 cm^2$ and a slope of 30 kPa/s was used (Algometer type II, SBMEDIC Electronics, 170 63 Solna, Sweden). PPT measurements are both reliable [196] and valid [197] for different regions of the spine [198, 199]. In healthy subjects the repeatability of PPT measurements is high, but also the inter-individual variation is high [195]. In study 3 PPT was measured at the same side and level of the wire insertion at the point of the zygapophysial joints. The mean of three consecutive measurements was taken for analysis after having discarded the first measure because this is reported to be higher than the following ones [200]. PPT at a reference point away from the painful cervical spine area like for example the tibialis anterior muscle has a predictive value in combination with sex and pain intensity in patients with neck pain following a whiplash injury [201]. A lower PPT at a point distant from the painful area is a clinical sign for widespread sensory hypersensitivity [202]. As no effect of an intervention on PPT was measured in study 3 and because general sensitization of the pain modulating system was present due to the chronicity of the patients' neck pain we abstained from assessing a reference point in order not to confound the main outcomes of the study by too many measurements with pain provocation.

3.5 VAS AND NDI (STUDIES 1-4)

In addition to the described EMG parameters, force and the PPT, the patients described their pain intensity on a visual analogue scale and their disability regarding different aspects of daily functioning completing the neck disability index.

3.5.1 Visual Analogue Scale (VAS)

The visual analogue scale (VAS) is usually a 10 cm long line with at the endpoints "no intensity/pain" and "worst possible/imaginable intensity/pain" [203]. There is no gold standard for the measurement of pain because it is a subjective variable and not an objective one [204]. The validity of the VAS therefore has been assessed by its correlation with other assessment tools like questionnaires and was found to be good [205, 206]. Reliability of the VAS is also difficult to assess because pain can change from one moment to another and consequently its measurement [207, 208]. The variability of successive assessments with the VAS can be up to 20% [203]. It is therefore recommended to use the mean of several measures over time to obtain reliable values [204]. For statistical analysis the VAS is considered a rational scale [209] and parametrical tests like t-test and ANOVA are appropriate [210, 211]. The VAS is more and more used in physiotherapy [212]. For a detailed review see Schomacher [213]. In conclusion, the VAS is a valid and reliable assessment tool for pain. The patients' pain intensity on the VAS was (mean ± SD) in study 2: 5.8 ± 1.6, in study 3: 6.1 ± 2.0, and in study 4: 5.4 ± 1.9.

3.5.2 Neck Disability Index (NDI)

The Neck Disability Index (NDI) is a 50-point index with 10 items assessing different aspects of daily functioning in patients with neck pain, each item scored on a 0 to 5 point scale [214]. The 10 items are divided into four groups regarding subjective symptoms (pain intensity, headache, concentration, sleeping), activities of daily living (lifting, work, driving, recreation), and discretionary activities of daily living (personal care, reading) [215, 216]. The NDI was first published in 1991 by Vernon and Mior [217]. It is considered a one-dimensional measure and can be interpreted as an interval scale [214]. The sum of the scores can be doubled to give a percentage score out of 100 (0-20 normal, 21-40 mild disability, 41-60 moderate, 61-80 severe and 80+ complete/exaggerated) [218]. In this project the simple sum was used as proposed in the original [216].

Like for the VAS the NDI is an evaluation of subjective parameters and no gold standard exists. Validity therefore can only be checked by the correlation to other assessment tools like the short form 36 health survey questionnaire, and it was found to be good [218-220]. The construct validity however was poor and the test-retest reliability was moderate, but due to the standardized questions the NDI is more appropriate for research than more individualized questionnaires like the Patient Specific Functional Scale [221]. In summary, the NDI is a widely used tool with good validity and acceptable reliability and is recommended for research in neck pain. The Neck Disability Index was (mean ± SD) in study 2: 21.2 ± 5.7, in study 3: 19.6 ± 7.5, and in study 4: 20.1 ± 6.8.

3.6 GENERAL PROCEDURE

After reviewing the inclusion and exclusion criteria, subjects were positioned prone. The PPT was measured in study 3. In all studies the spinous processes C2 and C7 were palpated and the insertion point(s) marked on the skin. The ultrasound transducer was placed transversally in the midline over the level of insertion and moved laterally to image the extensor muscles. After clear identification of the target muscle the skin was disinfected and needle insertion started. The correct location of the needle was checked by ultrasonography (Fig. 27), and the needle removed immediately leaving the wire in the muscle for the duration of the experiment.

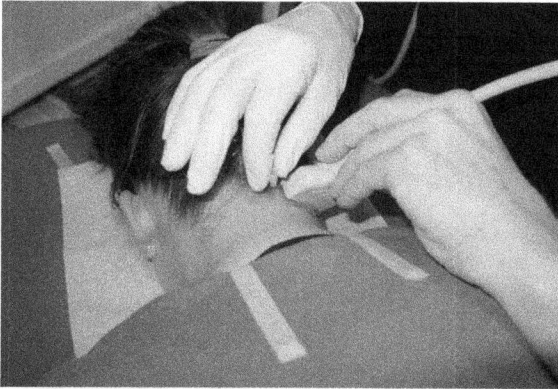

Fig. 27. Insertion of the carrier needle into semispinalis cervicis at level C3 guided by ultrasonography.

Subjects were then seated with their head rigidly fixed in the device for the measurement of multidirectional neck force (Fig. 28).

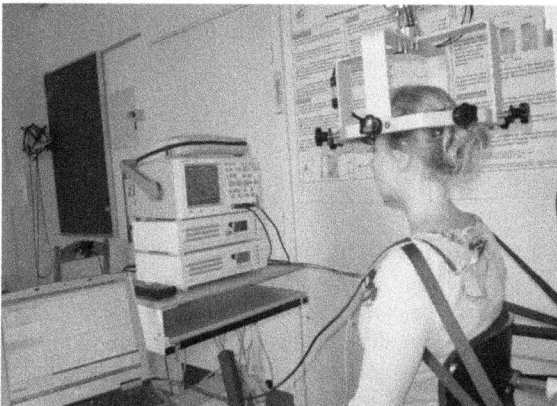

Fig. 28. The subject is sitting with the head fixed in the force device in front of the oscilloscope

The torso was fixed with straps to the seat back, knees and hips positioned in 90° of flexion and the hands resting on the laps. The force device measures force in the sagittal and coronal planes. Visual feedback was provided on the display of a force amplifier for the MVCs and for the circle contractions on an oscilloscope placed in front of the subject. Following a period of familiarization with the measuring device and a period to practice the desired contractions, subjects performed the motor tasks depending on the experiment and consisted of: static extension with MVC, submaximal ramp contractions, and circular contractions 0-360° at 15 and 30N over 12 s each.

In study 4 the patients performed static extension against manual resistances at the occiput and at the vertebral arches of C2 and C5 (Fig. 29). Visual feedback was provided on the computer screen. At the end of the experiment the wires were removed.

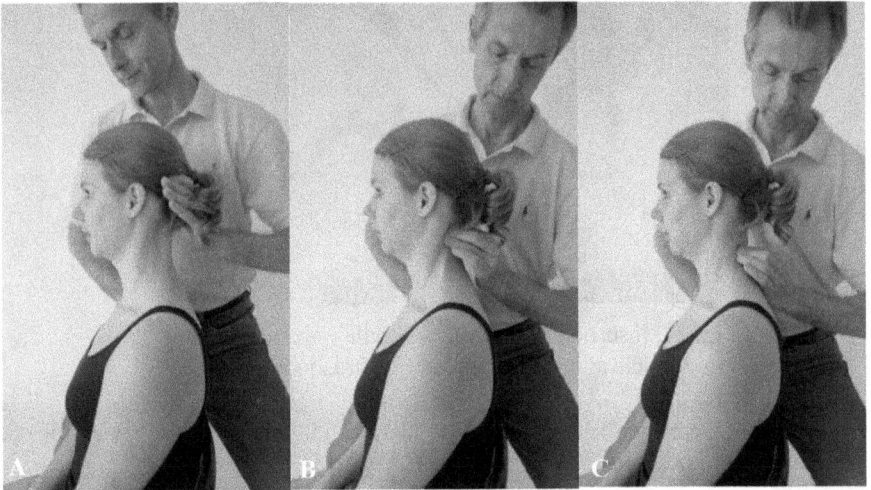

Fig. 29. Manual static resistances used in study 4while the patient is pushing backwards against a resistance at A) the occiput, and the vertebral arch of B) C2 and C) C5.

3.7 SIGNAL ANALYSIS

EMG signals were recorded in monopolar mode, i.e. the activation was measured between the different electrode in the muscle and two reference electrodes at the wrists representing the electrical zero-point. Monopolar electrodes record higher amplitude MUAPs which are slightly more complex, i.e. with more turns, than those registered with concentric electrodes [152]. The decomposition of the signal at low level contraction was used to analyze the single motor unit behaviour. The interference pattern was used to assess the mean EMG activity and to construct tuning curves for computing the directional specificity of the muscle's contraction (see also 1.8.4 and 3.3.3).

The raw EMG data collected in study 1 were decomposed with a decomposition algorithm (EMGlab), i.e. broken down into a sequence of action potentials from a single motor unit, the so-called motor unit action potential train (MUAPT) [161]. The raw EMG signals were pre-processed with a high-pass filter (1000 or 500 Hz) which reduces the amplitude of low frequencies (= noise reduction) [222]. All MUAPs above a set threshold amplitude were detected by the software and checked manually. Superimposed waveforms were resolved subtracting matching MUAPs one by one from the superimposed waveform [153]. Motor units that were active for less than half of the duration of the contraction and motor units with repeated inactive periods of several seconds were discarded from the analysis.

The average discharge rate and the discharge rate variability (coefficient of variation for interspike interval) were calculated from the decomposed data. Furthermore, the motor unit synchronization in the time (cross-correlation histograms) and frequency domain (coherence analysis) were computed for motor unit pairs within and across the two recording sites. The recruitment threshold (expressed as % of MVC) of each motor unit was estimated as the force level at which the motor unit began to discharge steadily (i.e., with separation between discharges in the range 20-200 ms) during the ramp contractions.

The interference EMG signals recorded in all 4 studies were analyzed by estimating the EMG amplitude as the average rectified value (ARV) of the signal in non-overlapping intervals of 300 ms (Study 1) or 250 ms (Studies 2-4).

3.7.1 Directional specificity

During the circular contractions, the amplitude of the intramuscular EMG was estimated as the average rectified value (ARV) of the signal in non-overlapping intervals of 250 ms. The ARV of the EMG as a function of the angle of force direction will be referred to in the following as directional activation curves [92]. The directional activation curves represent the modulation in intensity of muscle activity with the direction of force exertion and represent a closed area when expressed in polar coordinates (Fig. 30). The line connecting the origin with the central point of this area defined a directional vector, whose length was expressed as a percent of the mean ARV during the entire task [73]. This normalized vector length represents the specificity of muscle activation: it is equal to zero if the muscle is active in the same way in all directions and, conversely, it corresponds to 100% if the muscle is active in exclusively one direction. In addition, the EMG amplitude was averaged across the entire circular contraction to provide an indicator of the overall muscle activity.

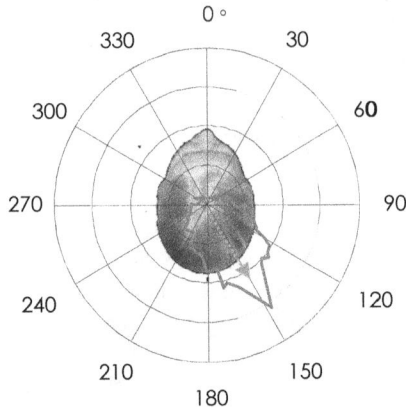

Fig. 30. Directional activation curve of semispinalis cervicis of a healthy subject obtained during a clockwise horizontal circle contraction at 15N measured at spinal level C2. The directional activation curve represents the modulation in intensity of muscle activity with the direction of force exertion. The central point of the tuning curve defined a directional vector (dashed arrow), whose length was expressed as a percent of the mean EMG average rectified value during the entire task.

3.8 STATISTICS

Analyses were computed with StatSoft. Inc. (2004). Statistica (data analysis software system), version 7. (www.statsoft.com). Data were checked for normality using the Kolmogorov-Smirnov test. Analysis of Variance (ANOVA) were used to analyze differences between different variables. Significant differences revealed by ANOVA were followed by post-hoc Student-Newman-Keuls (SNK) pair-wise comparisons. Pearson's correlation (r^2) was used in study 3 to look for an association between EMG activity (amplitude as well as directional specificity) of semispinalis cervicis and PPT at the spinal levels C2 and C5. Statistical significance was set at $P < 0.05$.

3.9 ETHICAL APPROVAL AND SIDE EFFECTS

Ethical approval for the studies was granted by the Regional Ethics Committee (N-20090039). All experiments were conducted respecting the declaration of Helsinki. In the studies of this thesis no infection and no incident was reported. No negative reactions were observed beside little skin bleeding for less than 1 min and slight soreness after needle insertion in a few subjects which quickly passed without any treatment and which is in line with the literature [67].

Chapter 4.

Results and discussions

Appendix 2 gives an overview of the results which are subsequently explained and discussed in detail.

4.1 STUDY 1

The first study investigated whether different fascicles of the semispinalis cervicis receive different synaptic input at a given external extension force according to their mechanical advantage and whether motor units innervating fascicles with a higher force demand during isometric neck extension would be recruited earlier. Intramuscular EMG was acquired at spinal levels C2 and C5 in 15 healthy subjects. They performed three sustained contractions into extension at 5%, 10% and 20% MVC and three ramp contractions from 0% to 30% MVC over 3 s. Signals were decomposed into single motor unit action potential trains (MUAPTs). In a second experiment the interference EMG was recorded in 8 healthy women during a ramp neck extension contraction from 0-50% MVC over 5 s. The MVC force for extension was 214.0 ± 45.0 N (mean $\pm$ SD) for the 7 healthy women and 259.1 ± 61.9 N for the 8 healthy men in the first experiment and 187.1 ± 46.1 N for the 8 healthy women in the second experiment.

4.1.1 Results

In the first experiment 98 motor units were identified across the three sustained contraction levels at C5 from 15 subjects, whereas only 18 motor units were detected in 5 of the 15 subjects at level C2. The analysis of the sustained contractions revealed a higher motor unit discharge rate at 20% MVC (C2: 13.25 ± 4.09 and C5: 13.80 ± 5.02) compared to 10% MVC (C2: 12.29 ± 1.91 and C5: 10.74 ± 4.03) and 5% MVC (C2: 11.3 ± 1.16 and C5: 9.41 ± 2.91) (P < 0.05) (Fig. 31). The discharge rate and the coefficient of variation of interspike intervals (ISI) were similar at levels C2 and C5 at all three force levels.

The short-term synchronization and the coherence analysis however were significantly higher within each spinal level than between both spinal levels indicating a different neural input to fascicles of the semispinalis cervicis at these levels for their independent control.

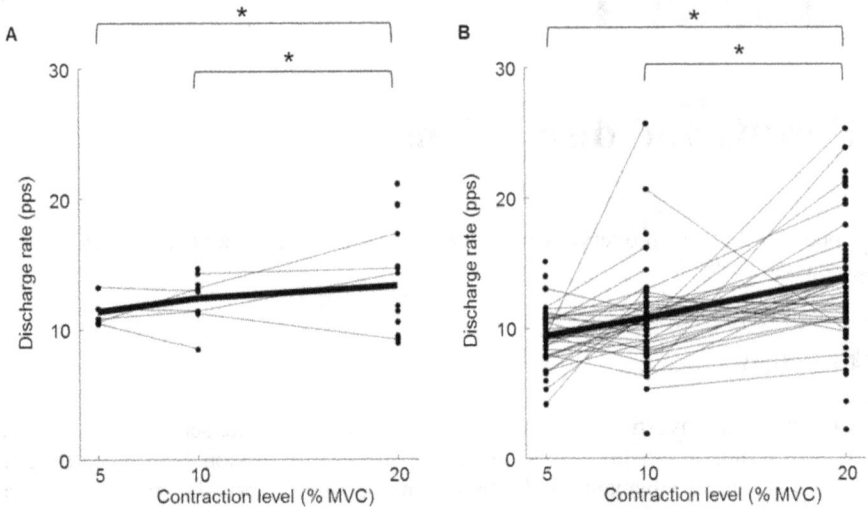

Fig. 31. The average discharge rate for all motor units identified at each contraction force for C2 (A) and C5 (B) respectively. The lines connect the discharge rates for those motor units that were identified at more than one force level. The bold lines represent the mean.

Significant peaks in the cross-histograms were found in 80% of the motor unit pairs (n = 307) when computed within the levels C2 and C5 (89.7% at C2 and 70.4% at C5, respectively). The level of synchronization of these motor unit pairs did not differ between levels (P = 0.91) (Fig. 32).

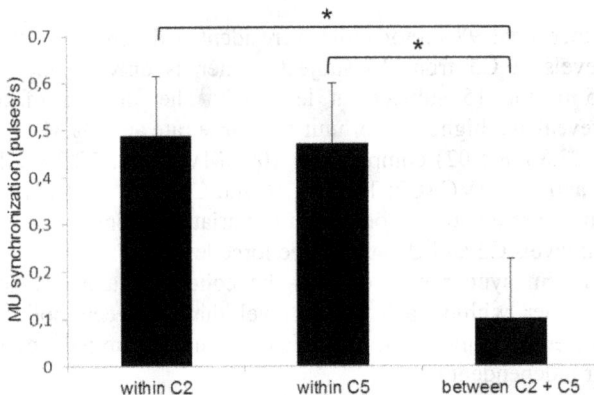

Fig. 32. Synchronization of motor unit pairs within each spinal level separately, and between both spinal levels. The level of synchronization was similar within spinal levels, but differed from the synchronization between both levels.

This indicates a common neural drive to the motor units within each spinal level. However, when computed between levels only 25% of the motor unit pairs (n = 110) presented significant peaks in the cross-histograms. Figure 33 shows representative data of one subject with absence of a clear peak in C for synchronization between C2 and C5 compared to the synchronization within levels C2 and C5 in A and B, respectively. Furthermore, the level of synchronization was significantly greater (P < 0.05) within levels (CIS = 0.48 ± 0.15 for C2; 0.47 ± 0.35 for C5), compared to pairs between levels (0.09 ± 0.07). This again indicates an independent neural drive to motor units at different spinal levels.

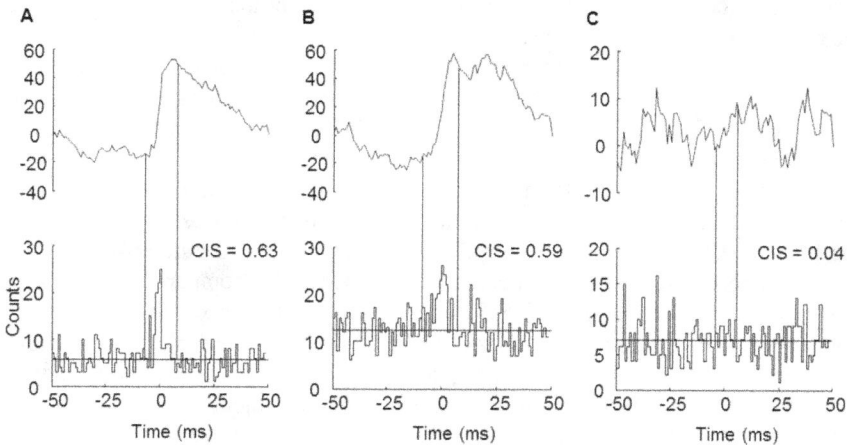

Fig. 33. Representative data showing the cross-histograms and cumulative sum (CuSum) for motor unit pairs in a representative subject during a 10% MVC contraction. The motor unit pairs are detected from the level C2 (A; CIS: 0.63), the level C5 (B; CIS: 0.59), and between the two levels (C; CIS: 0.04). The vertical lines indicate the boundaries of the synchronous peaks as determined from the CuSum. (CIS = Common Input Strength index)

The coherence in the frequency band 16-32 Hz was greater for motor unit pairs from the same level (0.17 ± 0.13 and 0.19 ± 0.19, respectively) than for motor pairs from different levels (0.04 ± 0.02) (P < 0.05). Significant coherence was found in 90% of the cases for motor unit pairs from the same level, but only in 29% of the cases for motor unit pairs from different levels. This further supports an independent neural drive to motor units at different spinal levels.

The ramp contractions showed a lower recruitment threshold at C5 (6.9 ± 4.3 % MVC) compared to C2 (10.3 ± 6.0 % MVC). This again points to a different neural drive to both spinal levels.

In the second experiment the mean amplitude of the interference EMG during the 0-50 % MVC ramps was 555.5 ± 364.0 μV at level C2 and 869.24 ± 388.35 μV at level C5. The normalized EMG amplitude was measured from intervals of 300 ms centred at the time instants of the ramp contractions corresponding to forces in the range 5% - 40% MVC, with 5% MVC increments. It increased with increasing force and was significantly different between each force level; $P < 0.0001$. Additionally, it was significantly greater for C5 than for C2 ($P < 0.05$) further supporting the independent neural drive to both spinal levels.

4.1.2 Discussion

The main finding of the study is the difference in the strength of synaptic input delivered to different fascicles of the semispinalis cervicis muscle during constant-force extensions. This may be partly due to the different mechanical advantage of the muscle fibers in different fascicles.

The discharge rates of the studied motor units were similar to those observed in other muscles [223-227]. The coefficient of variation for the interspike interval was also within the physiological range previously observed in other muscles (e.g., first dorsal interosseus, [224]).

The greater recruitment threshold for motor units at the C2 spinal level compared to C5 indicate that the net excitatory input to motoneurons innervating the fibers at C5 is greater than for C2 at a given force level. Furthermore, higher absolute interference EMG amplitude was detected at C5 compared to C2 during the ramped contraction from 0-50% MVC. Although it is difficult to make a comparison between global EMG amplitude and the number of detected motor units, which thus remain independent measures of muscle activity, both findings support an independent neural drive to fascicles of semispinalis cervicis at the two spinal levels.

A non-uniform activation of motor units within muscle regions as found in this study has also been observed in other human muscles, such as the extensor digitorum [228], the flexor digitorum profundus [229], the flexor digitorum superficialis [230], the upper trapezius muscle [226], and the external intercostal muscles [231, 232].

The analysis of the correlation between spike trains in the time and frequency domain indicated that the input to motoneurons innervating different fascicles of the semispinalis cervicis muscle is almost independent. The low degree of synchronization between pairs of motor units detected in the current study from two individual fascicles of the semispinalis cervicis muscle indicates a different neural input to semispinalis cervicis at these levels for their independent control. This is further supported by the observation that the coherence in the 16-32 Hz band was highest for pairs of motor units from the same fascicle of the semispinalis cervicis muscle.

The earlier recruitment of motor units in the caudal with respect to the cranial spinal segments can be explained by different moments exerted by the fascicles of the semispinalis cervicis muscle. Simple modeling allows a qualitative assessment of the distribution of forces for different fascicles. Fig. 34 shows a schematic model describing the mechanical action of the semispinalis cervicis fascicles during isometric extension of the head. In order to have equilibrium the external force has to be balanced by muscles and passive structures surrounding the cervical segments from C0 to C7.

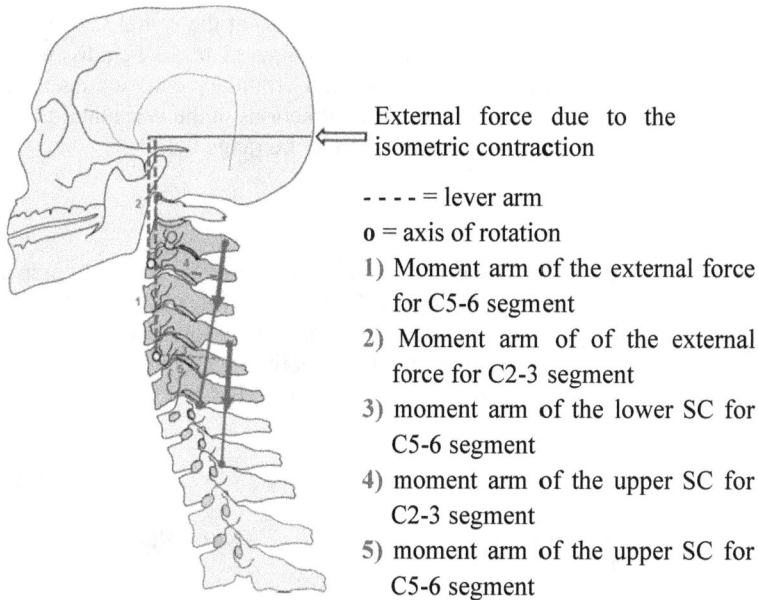

External force due to the
isometric contraction

- - - - = lever arm

o = axis of rotation

1) Moment arm of the external force
   for C5-6 segment

2) Moment arm of of the external
   force for C2-3 segment

3) moment arm of the lower SC for
   C5-6 segment

4) moment arm of the upper SC for
   C2-3 segment

5) moment arm of the upper SC for
   C5-6 segment

Fig. 34. Schematic representation of the moment system for the upper and
lower regions of the semispinalis cervicis (SC) during isometric neck
extension. The force moment of the reaction force of the head is greater for C5
than for C2. The required force to stabilize C5 is consequently higher than for
C2.

For example, the external moment to be balanced around C5-6 is larger than
the external moment around C2-3, due to the fact that the moment arm for the C5-6
segment (1) is larger than at C2-3 (2). So the fascicles spanning the joint C5-6 need
to create a higher extension moment than the fascicles spanning C2-3. These
conclusions are in agreement with the moment arms for extension of the different
fascicles of multifidus which decrease from ~1.4 to ~0.9 and to ~0.3 cm from C6-7
to C5-6 and C4-5, respectively, for the superficial fascicles, and from ~0.7 to ~0.6
and ~0.4 cm for the deep fascicles [131].

The lower recruitment threshold and consequently higher motor unit activation
at the spinal level C5 relative to C2 responds to the mechanical needs of the lower
cervical spine and the mechanical advantages of semispinalis cervicis fascicles at
this level. This highlights the importance of the muscle for movement control and
stabilization of the cervical spine and raises the question whether reduced
activation might be related to neck pain. The following study consequently
investigated the activation of semispinalis cervicis in patients with chronic neck
pain compared to healthy controls.

4.2 STUDY 2

In the second study the activity of semispinalis cervicis at the spinal level C3 was analysed in 10 women with chronic neck pain compared to 10 healthy women. Subjects performed two neck extension maximum voluntary contractions (MVC) separated by 1 min of rest followed by circle contractions in the horizontal plane at 15 and 30 N force with change in force direction in the range 0-360°.

4.2.1 Results

The maximum neck extension force was significantly lower in patients compared to controls (125.7 ± 55.2 N and 209.2 ± 56.9 N respectively; $P < 0.01$). Patients showed a significantly greater coefficient of variation of force compared to the control group during the circular contractions both at 15 and 30N (average; controls: 11.8 ± 1.7 %, patients: 14.8 ± 4.9 %; $F = 4.9$; $P < 0.05$) as illustrated by representative curves in Fig. 35.

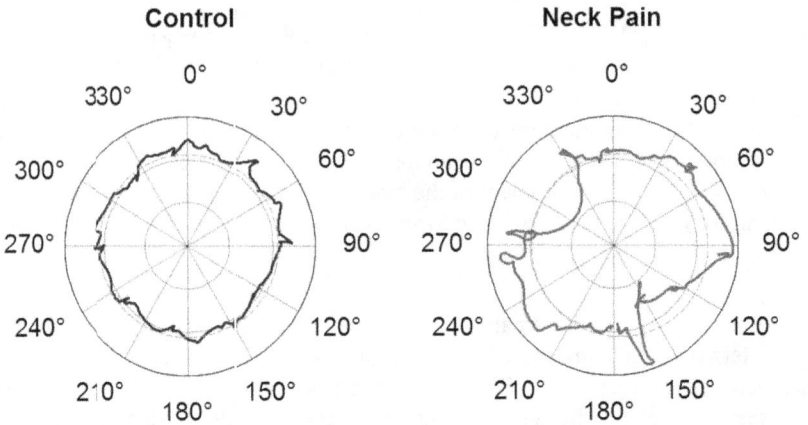

Fig. 35. Representative force traces obtained for a control subject and a patient performing a circular contraction at 15N in the counter-clockwise direction. In this example the coefficient of variation of force is 7.4 % and 17.5 % for the control and patient, respectively.

During isometric circle contractions from 0° to 360° at 15N and 30N in the horizontal plane the mean EMG amplitude was lower in patients compared to controls for both the 15N and 30N contractions (F = 10.5; P < 0.01) (Fig. 36).

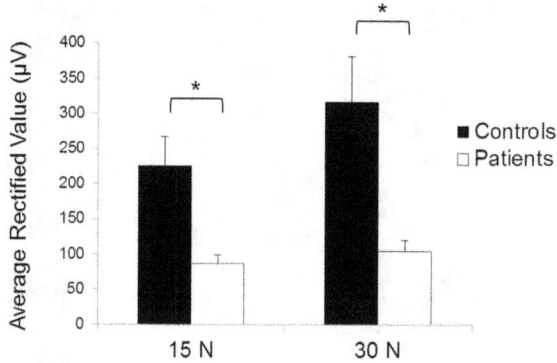

Fig. 36. Mean ± SE of the average rectified value of the intramuscular EMG of semispinalis cervicis muscle obtained during the circular contractions at both 15 and 30N of force for the patients with neck pain and control subjects. * = P < 0.001

The directional specificity of semispinalis cervicis is clearly seen in the representative directional activation curve of a control subject with the highest amplitude of activity towards ipsilateral posterolateral extension (Fig. 37). The representative activation curve of a patient however displayed more even activation levels of the semispinalis cervicis muscle for all directions.

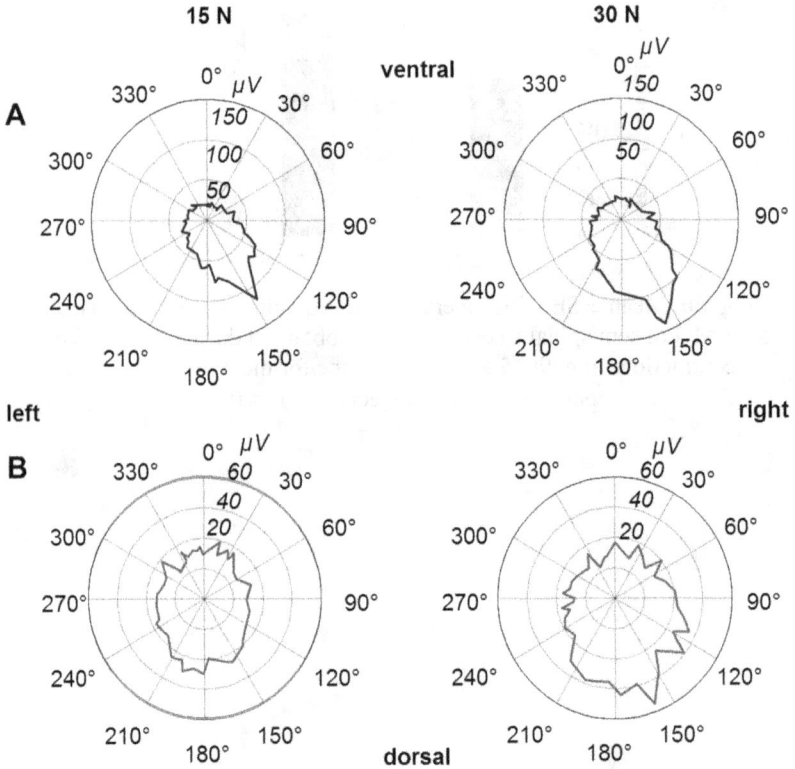

Fig. 37. Representative directional activation curves for a control subject (A) and a patient (B) performing circular contractions at 15 N and 30 N of force.

In the patient group, the directional specificity was significantly lower for both the 15N and 30N circular contractions compared to the controls (F = 4.7; P < 0.05) (Fig. 38). Nevertheless, the average of directional specificity across groups was higher at 30N contractions compared to 15N contractions (average across groups: 23.0 ± 9.8 % and 28.9 ± 10.4 % for the 15N and 30N contractions respectively; F = 5.2; P < 0.05).

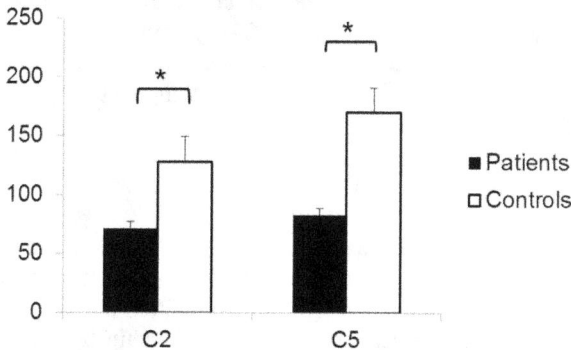

Fig. 38. Mean $\pm$ SE of the directional specificity in the intramuscular EMG of the semsispinalis cervicis muscle obtained during the circular contractions at both 15 and 30 N of force for the patients with neck pain and control subjects. * = P < 0.05

4.2.2 Discussion

The results showed that, contrary to asymptomatic individuals, the semispinalis cervicis muscle has reduced and less defined activity during a multidirectional isometric contraction in patients with chronic neck pain. Reduced activation of the semispinalis cervicis may impact on support of the cervical spine which could be relevant for the maintenance and perpetuation of neck pain.

For the control subjects the activity of the semispinalis cervicis muscle was tuned selectively for the direction of force, i.e. the muscle was active predominately in extension with a small ipsilateral component. Patients with neck pain however showed reduced specificity of semispinalis cervicis activity as has also been observed for the sternocleidomastoid and splenius capitis muscles in patients with chronic neck pain [73, 92]. This loss of directional specificity is interpreted as an attempt to stiffen the cervical spine similar to co-activation of cervical muscles [103, 233, 234]. However reduced specificity of both the sternocleidomastoid and splenius capitis was associated with an overall increase in activity in patients with neck pain [73, 92]. The opposite was observed for the semispinalis cervicis muscle in this study. This finding is in accordance with observations from the deep cervical flexor muscles, the longus colli and longus capitis, which also show reduced activity in patients with chronic neck pain of idiopathic and traumatic origin [20].

A recent study has found lower activity of semispinalis cervicis and multifidus in patients with mechanical neck pain at levels C5-6 and C7-T1, but not at level C2-C3 during cervical extension with the head in neutral position [98]. In a similar study pain was experimentally induced in healthy subjects injecting hypertonic saline into the upper trapezius muscle which results in lower activation of multifidus and semispinalis cervicis at C7-T1 but not at C2-3 level [124]. Interestingly, splenius capitis showed reduced activation on the side of pain at the level C7-T1 which was close to the injection but higher activation on the opposite side at level C2-3 [124]. However, in these studies measurements were made with mfMRI and the exercise was made in prone lying which can be assumed to stimulate the extensor muscles in a different way than the exercise in sitting position used in the current study.

The lower activity of semispinalis cervicis identified at C3 raises the question whether it is a local or a generalized phenomenon. Central and peripheral sensitisation of the nervous system might influence EMG activity and can partially be assessed by pressure pain sensitivity. The relationship between pressure pain sensitivity and level of activation of the semispinalis cervicis musle was therefore addressed in study 3.

4.3 STUDY 3

In this study 10 female patients with chronic neck pain and 10 matched healthy women were investigated. The PPT was recorded over the zygapophyseal joints C2 and C5. At these levels EMG activity and the directional specificity of semispinalis cervicis were measured during horizontal circle contractions from 0° to 360° at 15N and 30N.

4.3.1 Results

The PPT was significantly lower in patients at both levels (C2: 71.4 ± 34.5 kP; C5: 83.1 ± 38.7 kPa) compared to controls (C2: 128.0 ± 43.4 kP; C5: 169.9 ± 57.4 kP; $P < 0.01$; Fig. 39). Across both groups the PPT were lower at C2 compared to C5 ($P < 0.001$).

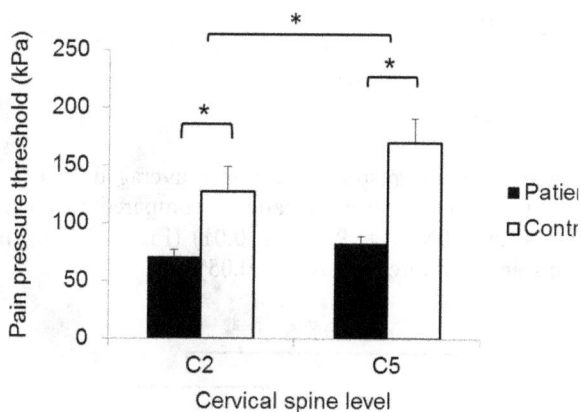

Fig. 39. Pressure pain thresholds of patients and controls at spinal levels C2 and C5. * = P < 0.05

The EMG amplitude and directional specificity were lower in patients compared to controls without any difference between the spinal levels and force levels (Table 1).

Table. 1. Mean and standard deviation of the mean EMG activity (μV) and directional specificity of semispinalis cervicis during the horizontal circle contractions.

		Mean EMG activity (μV) ± SD		Directional specificity ± SD	
		15N	30N	15N	30N
C2	Controls	155.34 ± 70.28	180.05 ± 85.48	19.96 ± 14.06	25.13 ± 14.53
	Patients	121.07 ± 62.07	110.61 ± 39.02	18.87 ± 7.88	20.74 ± 7.22
C5	Controls	162.03 ± 52.01	195.22 ± 64.31	25.28 ± 13.85	30.33 ± 14.72
	Patients	136.95 ± 53.09	143.04 ± 63.57	16.69 ± 7.24	17.91 ± 9.25

The EMG activity of semispinalis cervicis averaged across the circular contractions was significantly lower in patients compared to controls for both contractions at 15N and 30N (F = 9.7; P < 0.01) (Fig. 40). No difference was observed between spinal and force levels (P > 0.05).

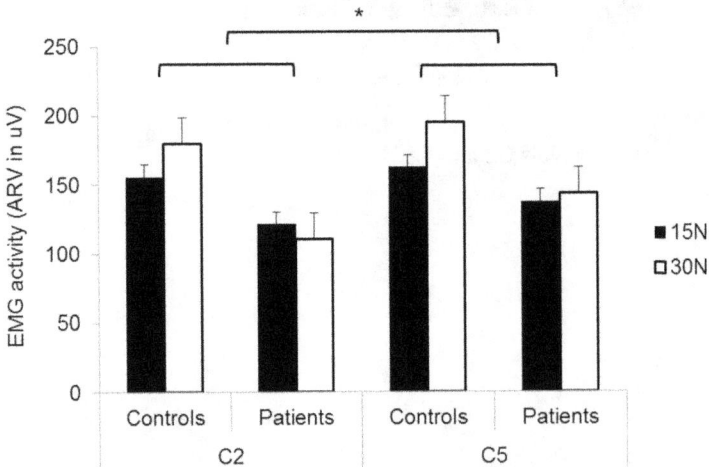

Fig. 40. Mean ± SE of the mean EMG activity (average rectified value = ARV) of the semispinalis cervicis muscle of healthy controls and patients performing a circular contraction in the horizontal plane at 15N and 30N with change in force direction in the range 0-360°. * = P < 0.05

Figure 41 shows representative directional activation curves of semispinalis cervicis recorded at both C2 and C5 during a circular contraction performed at 15N for a control and a patient. The control subject shows well-defined directional specificity. The patient with neck pain on the contrary presents with almost constant activity in all directions.

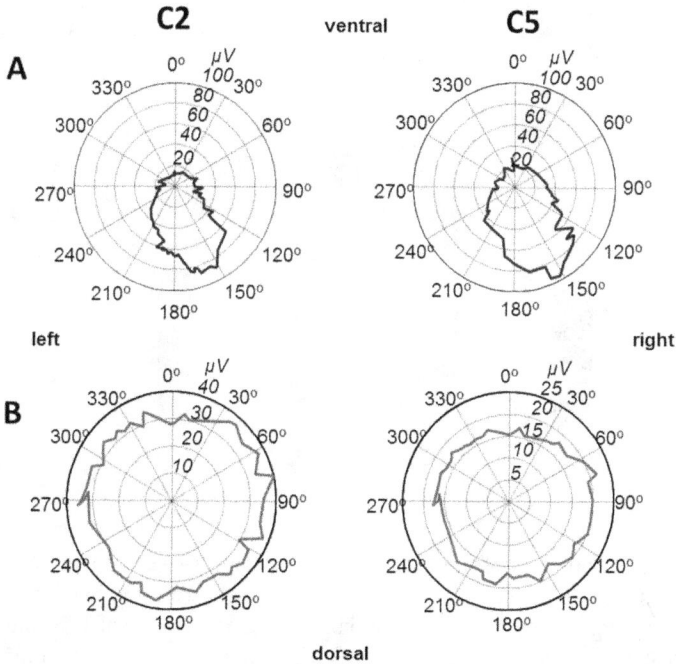

Fig. 41. Representative directional activation curves of semispinalis cervicis muscle at the spinal levels C2 and C5 for a 15 N contraction during a clockwise circular contraction for a control subject and a patient with neck pain.

The directional specificity was significantly different for patients compared to controls for both the 15N and 30N circular contractions (F = 6.17; P < 0.05) as expressed by the vector length (Fig. 42). The vector length is expressed as a percent of the mean ARV during the entire task: 100% means that the EMG amplitude is different from zero in exclusively one direction (ideal specificity). No difference was observed between spinal and force levels (P > 0.05).

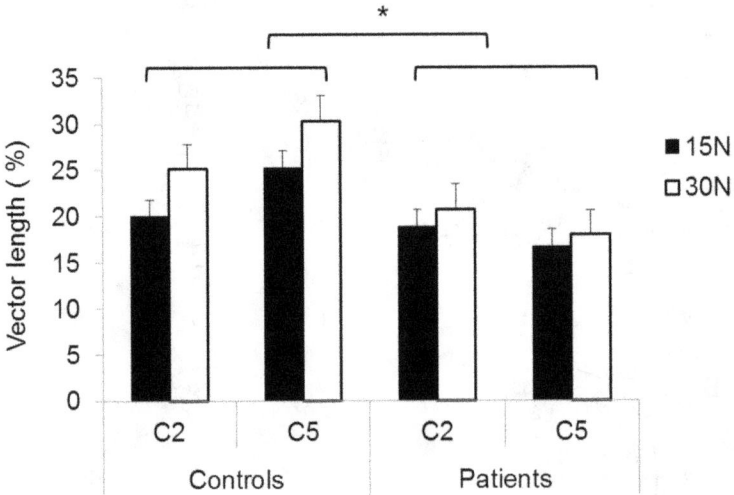

Fig. 42. Mean ± SE of the directional specificity (= vector length) of the semispinalis cervicis muscle of healthy controls and patients performing a circular contraction in the horizontal plane at 15N and 30N with change in force direction in the range 0-360°. * = P < 0.05

A significant correlation was identified between the PPT and directional specificity of semispinalis cervicis activity ($R^2 = 0.22$, $P < 0.05$; Fig. 43a) and between PPT and mean EMC activity ($R^2 = 0.15$, $P < 0.05$; Fig. 43b). The mean activity of the semispinalis cervicis and directional specificity were also significantly correlated ($R^2 = 0.41$, $P < 0.05$; Fig. 43c.).

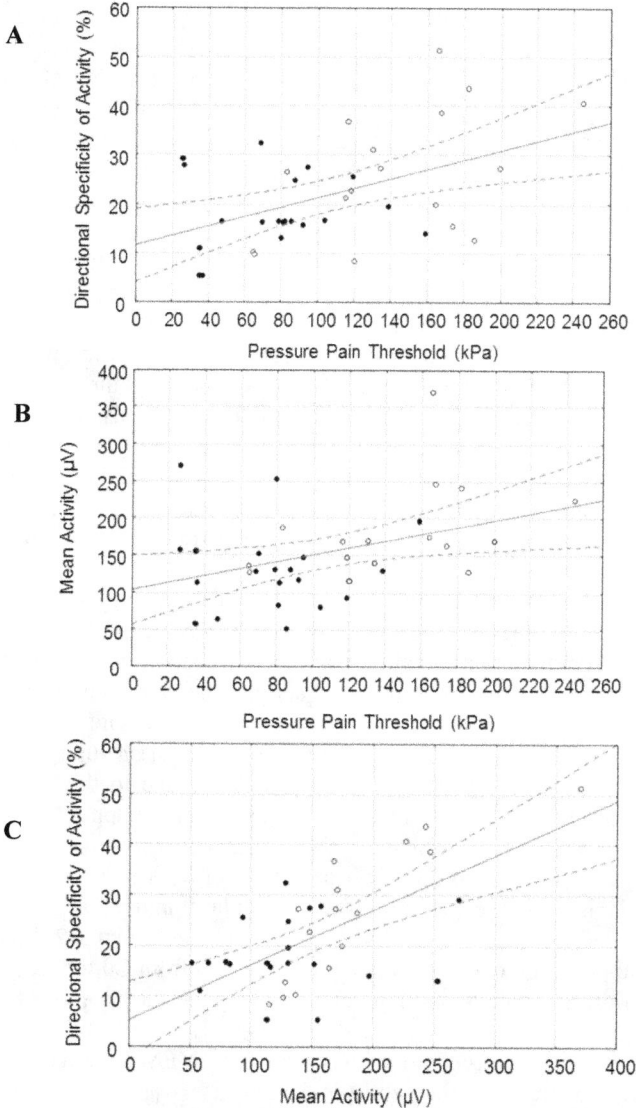

Fig. 43. Scatter plot showing the correlation between A) the PPT and directional specificity, B) PPT and EMG activity of semispinalis cervicis activity, and C) directional specificity and mean EMG activity. Dashed lines represent the 95% confidence interval. (O = controls / ● = patients)

4.3.2 Discussion

The PPT over the C2 and C5 zygapophyseal joints was significantly lower in women with chronic neck pain compared to controls which is consistent with previous observations in patients with neck pain over zygapophyseal joints [235] and neck muscles [236]. At the same spinal levels patients showed lower EMG amplitude and lower directional specificity of the semispinalis cervicis during the multidirectional isometric contractions of the neck. This is in line with the findings observed for the semispinalis cervicis muscle when measured at C3 in study 2. Lower activity of the semispinalis cervicis (and multifidus) as measured with mfMRI was also found in patients with mechanical neck pain when assessed at C5-6 and C7-T1 during cervical extension [98] and at C7-T1 in healthy subjects with experimental pain in the upper trapezius [124] but not at level C2-3. The observation of altered activation of the semispinalis cervicis muscle across different spinal levels suggests that it is a generalised phenomenon in patients with neck pain rather than being localised to a specific segment. Some studies have shown site specific changes in muscle structure which can occur uniquely at painful segments of the spine [192, 193] although other studies demonstrate widespread changes in muscle composition which are not isolated to one level of the spine. For example, fatty infiltration of the neck extensors in patients with persistent whiplash-induced neck pain is observed across all vertebral levels (C3-7) (Elliott et al 2006). The most painful segment was not specifically identified in this current study and therefore further investigations are required to reveal the extent or distribution patterns of altered EMG activity across differing spinal levels with respect to the painful segments.

As a general finding the PPT over the zygapophyseal joint at C2 was lower than at C5 in both groups. This suggests that, in general, C2 is more sensitive to mechanical stimulation or palpation than C5. This substantiates that PPT measures the tenderness of the tissues to pressure and not the pain complaint by the patient [195]. Indeed, only a weak correlation has been shown between PPT over the cervical spinous process and subacute neck pain after a whiplash injury [237]. It has been proposed that C2 may be more sensitive to loads due to the mechanical stress caused by the encounter of the movement coupling of the upper (C0 to C3) and the lower (C2 to C7) cervical spine [238]. The sensitivity and vulnerability of the C2 segment may contribute to the frequent reports of neck pain in this area [2, 47]. For example, in half of the patients after a whiplash injury which complained of headache, the source of pain was the zygapophyseal joint C2 [47]. Additionally, mechanical palpation over the zygapophyseal joints from C0 to C4, but not C5-C7, was significantly more painful in patients with headache compared to healthy controls [61].

Evidence of a correlation between PPT and EMG activity and PPT and directional specificity of the semispinalis cervicis was found when patient and control data were pooled. However, PPT was only weakly correlated to EMG activity and directional specificity of semispinalis cervicis, suggesting that other factors may contribute to this finding. For example, general psychological distress and fear avoidance behaviour have a strong influence on movement and motor control [71]. To date, few studies have examined correlations between PPT and EMG activity in patients with pain. A weak correlation for example was found between masseter and sternocleidomastoid PPT and EMG activity in patients with tenderness during palpation of the masseter muscle [200].

Lower EMG activity in the semispinalis cervicis muscle in the presence of lower PPT might be explained by the pain adaptation model which suggests inhibition of muscles due to pain in order to avoid movement for protection of painful muscles and/or joints [239]. This theory is supported by several experimental studies [240-243]. The positive correlation between lower EMG activity of semispinalis cervicis and the lower PPT in the current study cannot consequently be explained by pain alone but may be influenced by central and peripheral sensitisation of the nervous system.

In consideration of the observation of reduced activity of semispinalis cervicis in patients with neck pain an exercise to enhance the activation of this muscle would seem relevant for patients with neck pain. Typical exercises for the neck extensors utilize resistance either from the weight of the head or by external forces like pulleys applied to the head [16, 19, 244]. These exercises activate all extensor muscles [100] and are therefore not specific to target the deeper neck extensor muscles [27]. Study 4 was therefore conducted to investigate three exercises in order to determine which if any are able to emphasize the activation of the semispinalis cervicis muscle.

4.4 STUDY 4

Ten patients with chronic neck pain were included in this study and performed isometric contractions into neck extension at the individual maximal intensity against manual resistance of the therapist applied at a) the occiput and at the vertebral arch of b) C2 and c) C5. The ratio between the activation of the semispinalis cervicis and splenius capitis was assessed to determine which exercise was best at obtaining relative isolation of the semispinalis cervicis muscle.

4.4.1 Results

The absolute ARV (μV) showed higher activity of semispinalis cervicis muscle with the resistance at C2 and an overall higher activity with the resistance at the occiput (Fig. 44). However, the manual resistance could not be standardized across conditions thus statistical tests were not performed on this data.

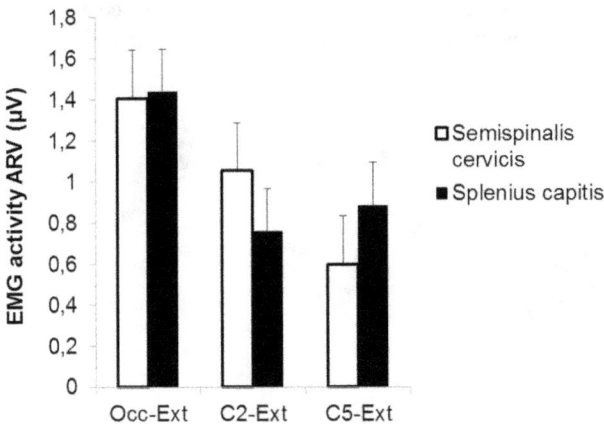

Fig. 44. Mean and standard error of the EMG average rectified values (μV) of semispinalis cervicis and splenius capitis muscle during the three isometric contractions into extension with resistance at the occiput, at C2, and at C5.

The ratio of the EMG activity of semispinalis cervicis and splenius capitis was therefore computed which eliminates the bias of variation in manual resistance. This ratio of EMG ARV showed a relatively increased activation of semispinalis cervicis compared to splenius capitis with resistance at C2 (2.53 ± 2.43 µV) compared to the resistance at the occiput (1.39 ± 1.00 µV) and C5 (1.16 ± 0.85 µV) (Fig. 45).

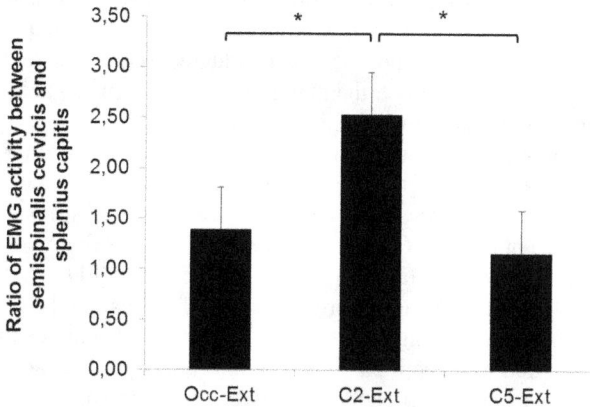

Fig. 45. Mean and standard error of the ratio of semispinalis cervicis and splenius capitis EMG ARV (µV) during manual resistance applied at three different locations as the patients produced an extension force (* = P < 0.05).

The main effect of a one-way ANOVA for the location of resistance was significant (F = 5.04; P = 0.018) with differences between the occiput versus C2 (P = 0.024) and C5 versus C2 (P = 0.022), but not between the occiput and C5 (P = 0.625) in the post-hoc Student-Newman-Keuls (SNK) pair-wise comparisons.

4.4.2 Discussion

The results of this study indicate that an accentuated activation of semispinalis cervicis is possible pushing against an external resistance applied at the vertebral arch cranial to the target muscle. The results confirm that a muscle with insertions at the spine such as the semispinalis cervicis is better suited to resist an external force applied at the spine compared to a muscle inserting at the occiput like splenius capitis.

Isometric head/neck extension at 20% of the maximum voluntary contraction performed in 15° of craniocervical extension increased only the activity of semispinalis capitis muscle at levels C2 and C5 and of multifidus and semispinalis cervicis at level C7 compared to the exercise performed in neutral position in healthy subjects [245]. Compared to healthy controls, patients with mechanical neck pain showed less activity of multifidus and semispinalis cervicis muscles at levels C5-6 and C7-T1 but not at C2-3, and of splenius capitis muscle at C7-T1 during cervical static extension in prone lying, while other cervical extensors did not differ between both groups [98]. This was only found in a craniocervical neutral position but not in 15° of craniocervical extension and might indicate that prepositioning of the head does not result in selected activation of cervical extensors. Lower activity of the deep cervical extensors was also found at the level C7-T1 but not at C2-3 in healthy subjects with experimental pain in the upper trapezius [124]. Both these studies were conducted with muscle functional magnetic resonance images for which the magnitude of T2 shift required to justify clinical significance is still not known as stated by the authors [98].

The increased activation of semispinales cervicis at C3 by a direct manual resistance at C2 but not at C5 might be explained by the anatomical configuration of the muscle. The fibres of semispinalis cervicis inserting at C2 are best suited to resist an external force applied at C2 and were recorded by the fine wire electrode located at C3 (Fig. 46b). A resistance applied at the occiput (Fig. 46a) or at C5 (Fig. 46c) requires activity of the recorded fibres of semispinalis cervicis for stiffening the spine assuming a single axis of rotation at C7-T1, but not for directly counteracting the externally applied force. Consequently, the activation of semispinalis cervicis was not significantly increased relative to splenius capitis.

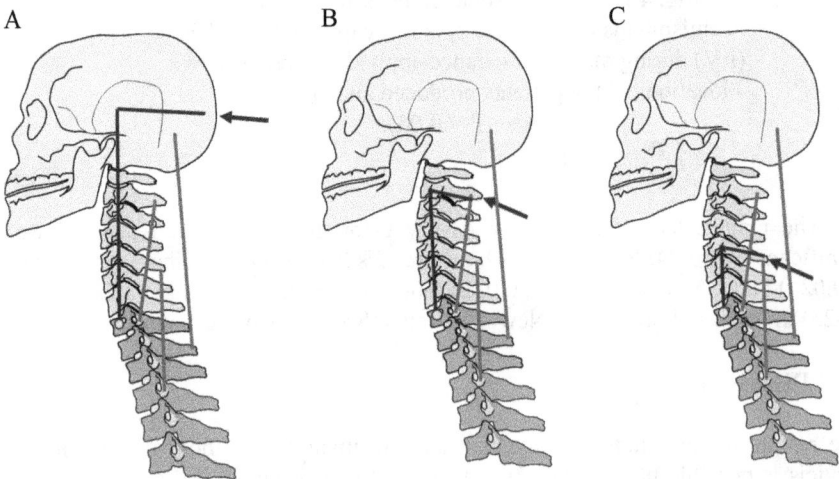

Fig. 46 Simplified illustration of the three manual resistances (arrows) at A) the occiput, B) the vertebral arch of C2, and C) the vertebral arch of C5 with a common movement axis at segment C7-T1 and the assumption that other muscles stiffen all other spinal segments.

Splenius capitis is best suited to act on the angle lever of the occiput (a), while the muscle fibres of semispinalis cervicis inserting on C2 act best on the angle lever C2 (b) and the fasicles inserting on to C5 on the angle lever of C5 (c). A similar analysis would be necessary for all other axes of rotation of the cervical spine for a comprehensive exploration of the system. However, this explanation remains hypothetical because the manual contact at the level of the vertebral arch is not directly onto the vertebra but rather through the muscles and is not limited to one single level (Fig. 47). The tactile stimulation of the skin and the muscles by the finger pressure might influence the activation of the muscles. Further research is necessary to investigate the mechanisms of muscle activation by manual resistance. Less invasive techniques like muscle functional magnetic resonance imaging [245] and tissue velocity ultrasound imaging (TVI) [138] might facilitate the search for the best exercise for activation of the deep cervical extensors in the future.

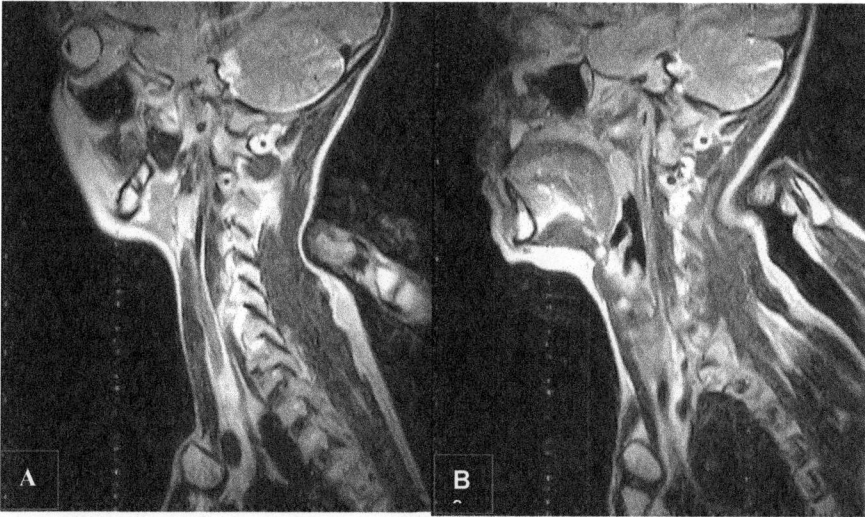

Fig. 47 MRI scan of a 39 year old healthy female showing the researchers thumb (A) and index finger (B) pushing with the maximal tolerable force on the vertebral arch of about C3. (from: Schomacher and Learman, 2010; with permission from the publisher)

Chapter 5.

General discussion

This thesis investigated the neural drive to semispinalis cervicis muscle in healthy subjects and in patients with chronic neck pain and examined whether various exercises could selectively activate the semispinalis cervicis muscle. The main findings are:

Study 1: A non-uniform single motor unit behaviour and a partly independent synaptic input to different fascicles of semispinalis cervicis muscle as seen by less motor unit synchronization between two spinal levels, a lower recruitment threshold at level C5 compared to C2 and consequently a higher number of recruited MUs with bigger global EMG amplitude at C5 compared to C2 during the static head extension task.

Study 2: A significantly lower activity and directional specificity of semispinalis cervicis at C3 in patients with chronic neck pain compared to healthy controls during a multidirectional isometric contraction.

Study 3: Significantly lower PPT over C2 and C5 zygapophyseal joints in women with chronic neck pain compared to controls and lower EMG amplitude and lower directional specificity of the semispinalis cervicis at the same spinal levels during a multidirectional isometric contraction. PPT of patients and controls together showed a significant, albeit weak, correlation with EMG mean activity and directional specificity of semispinalis cervicis suggesting a possible association between pressure pain sensitivity and reduced muscle activity.

Study 4: Higher activation of the semispinalis cervicis relative to the splenius capitis at the level of C3 when pushing against a manual resistance applied at the vertebral arch of C2 compared to the same exercise with resistance at the occiput or at C5.

The spine is a complex system consisting of several functional units working together. Its high mobility is at the expense of stability. Abnormal large intervertebral motions are considered a main origin of mechanical pain by causing either compression and/or stretching of inflamed neural elements or abnormal deformation of passive spinal structures like ligaments, joint capsules, annular fibres, and end-plates [246]. This can be avoided by maintaining the vertebrae within the neutral zone, i.e. the region of high flexibility or laxity around the neutral position [54]. In order to achieve this the body uses the passive elements of the spinal column including ligaments, disc, and joint facet orientation, the active spinal muscles and the neural control unit [246]. Muscles able to control movements of single segments are those with insertions directly onto the vertebrae [134]. For the cervical spine these are the deep cervical flexors and extensors which together create a muscular sleeve enclosing and stabilizing the cervical spine [99]. The performance of these muscles is adapted in different ways at different spinal levels since the mechanical stress acting on the cervical spine is not distributed homogeneously. Movements of the head for example during whiplash trauma provoke major stress in the lower cervical spine due the lever arm of the head which is longer at this point than in the middle and upper cervical region with facet joint lesions occurring mostly in the C5-C6 and C6-C7 segments [52, 55]. Movements of the segment C2-3 comprise high stress due to the encounter of the movement coupling from the upper cervical spine (C0 to C3) and the lower one (C2 to C7) in this segment [238, 247]. This might explain frequent occurrence of pain in the C2-3 segment [2, 47]. It can be supposed that the neural drive to the stabilizing muscles at these different spinal levels is not homogeneously distributed but according to the mechanical needs of the spine which varies in regions of the cervical spine.

This hypothesis was investigated in the first study by analysing the behaviour of motor units of the semispinalis cervicis at the spinal levels C2 and C5 in healthy subjects during an isometric extension task. The recruitment threshold of motor units was lower and more motor units were activated at C5 compared to C2. This responds to the mechanical needs of the cervical spine which are higher in its lower part compared to its middle and upper one, and to the larger and consequently anatomically more advantageous moment arms of the lower fascicles compared to the upper ones. Neural input to muscles following mechanical needs and advantages has already been described in extremity [226, 228-230 248, 249] and intercostal muscles [231, 232, 250-252]. These neurophysiological properties of the semispinalis cervicis in addition to its anatomical characteristics suggest that this muscle is able to resist different forces acting on the cervical spine and might therefore be important for motor control and stabilization of the cervical spine. It was hypothesized that the activity of this muscle is reduced in patients with neck pain.

This hypothesis was analysed in the second and third study by measuring the EMG activity of semispinalis cervicis at the level of C2, C3 and C5 in patients with chronic neck pain and healthy controls during isometric circular contractions in the horizontal plane. Both studies showed that the EMG amplitude of the semispinalis cervicis was lower in patients which is in line with similar findings in the deep cervical flexors [20, 86, 87]. The directional specificity of semispinalis cervicis activity was also lower in patients, i.e. its ability to contract in well-defined preferred directions according to its anatomical position relative to the spine. Loss of directional specificity of activity has also been observed for the sternocleidomastoid and splenius capitis muscles in patients with neck pain [73, 92].

Pain may result in a inhibition of the agonist muscle such as the semispinalis cervicis during neck extension to limit the activity of the painful muscle and movement [239]. This pain adaptation theory is supported by growing evidence [240-243] with several variations depending on the mechanical action of the task performed (for references see: [253]). Sensitization of the nervous system might be a further factor influencing EMG activity of the deep semispinalis cervicis muscle. The correlation between PPT and EMG activity and directional specificity however was only weak. This might indicate that in addition to pain and tenderness of the tissues to pressure there might be other explanations for reduced EMG activity and directional specificity like for example simple disuse as a consequence of fear of pain. The observation of altered activation of the semispinalis cervicis muscle across different spinal levels suggests that it is a generalised phenomenon in patients with neck pain. However, since the symptomatic segment was not localized it cannot be excluded that EMG activity and directional specificity were lower at the symptomatic segment of each individual patient and not in general and that this effect was "washed out" by computing the mean values.

5.1 FUNCTIONAL AND STRUCTURAL CHANGES IN THE CERVICAL MUSCLES RELATED TO PAIN

The cause-effect relationships between functional and structural changes in the cervical muscles and neck pain are poorly understood [242]. Functional changes in muscle activity reflect altered neuromuscular control of movement and stability of the cervical spine. Structural changes of the muscles associated with neck pain might be a consequence or a cause of these functional changes.

Pain might inhibit muscle contraction in order to avoid the painful movement [239]. This might explain lower activation of the deep cervical flexors [20, 21] and extensors as shown in this thesis and in a recent study [98] in patients with chronic neck compared to healthy controls. The superficial cervical flexors [20, 21, 88] and cervical extensors [93, 97, 254] on the other hand show increased activity in patients with neck pain which might be caused by nociceptor induced increased activity in the gamma motor neurons leading to increased activity and muscle stiffness [255]. Patients with neck pain also show increased co-activation observed for the splenius capitis [73] and sternocleidomastoid muscle [73, 92] which may be an attempt to better control movement and stabilize the cervical spine in the presence of pain induced deep muscle dysfunction [21, 80, 234].

In addition or as a result of altered muscle activation several outcomes of muscle performance are affected in patients with neck pain such as strength [71], endurance [77], range of motion [256], altered proprioception [257], and reduced head-eye-coordination [69, 148, 258].

Pain probably does not have a direct effect on the muscle fibres, but part of the normal response to pain and associated psychological stress is the activation of the sympathetic nervous system with an increase of adrenaline and vasoconstriction which affects the removal of metabolic by-products like lactic acid during muscle contraction [179]. Physiological sympathetic activation elicited by the cold pressor test for example generally alters muscle contractility [259] and resulted in increased activity of the sternocleidomastoid and splenius muscle in healthy volunteers [260]. Also mental stress such as computer work increases the activation of upper trapezius [261]. These and similar factors may influence the contractile mechanism of the muscles indirectly by pain [242]. Structural changes might follow injury or longstanding altered motor control strategies as described above. The structural changes include for example biochemical alterations of muscle tissue such as higher serotinin (5-HT) and glutamate in the upper trapezius of women with work related myalgia [262], fat infiltration after whiplash injury in the deep cervical flexors [107] and extensors [108], muscle atrophy reflected by lower cross-sectional area of the deep cervical flexors [107] and extensors [112], and fibre transformation from type I to type II in several cervical muscles[120]. For a detailed review of structural and functional changes in muscles due to neck pain see Falla and Farina 2008 and 2007 [57, 242].

It is unknown whether functional changes induce or follow structural changes in the muscle and likely there is an interactive relationship between functional and structural changes (Fig. 48).

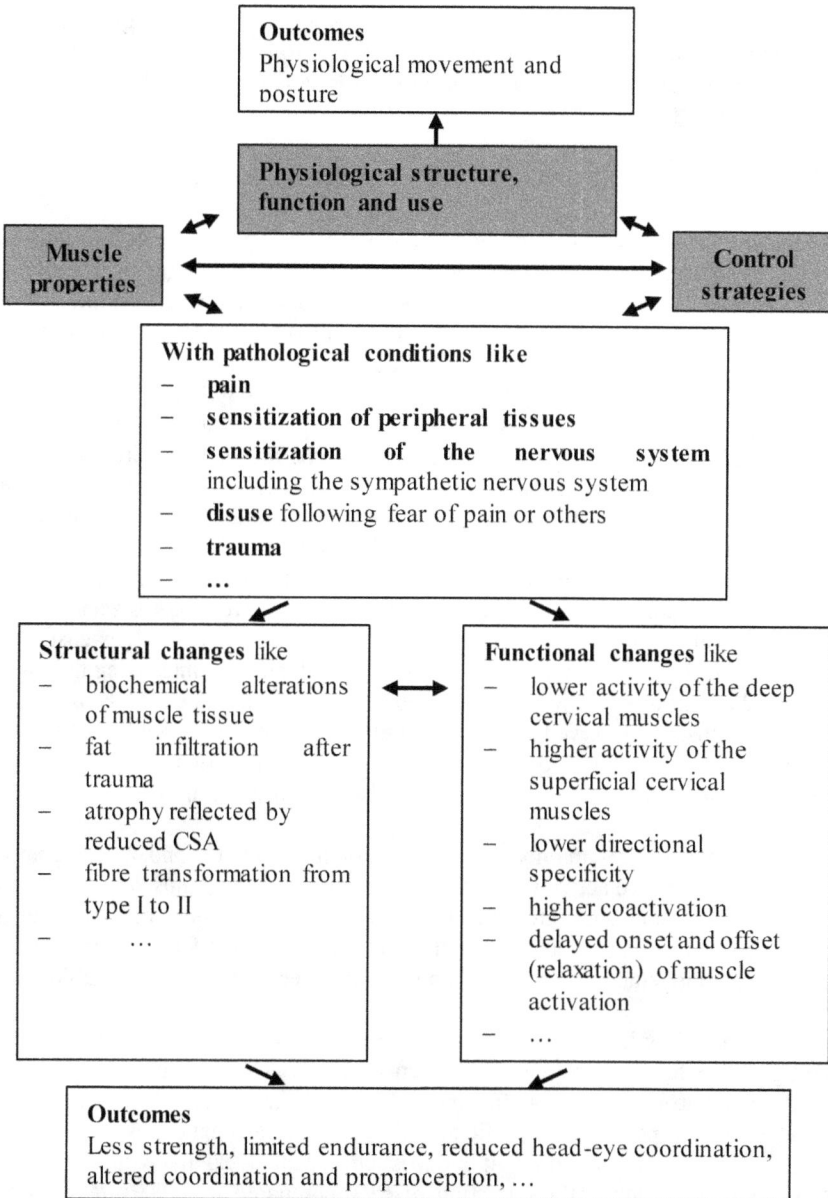

Outcomes
Physiological movement and posture

Physiological structure, function and use

Muscle properties

Control strategies

With pathological conditions like
– **pain**
– **sensitization of peripheral tissues**
– **sensitization of the nervous system** including the sympathetic nervous system
– **disuse** following fear of pain or others
– **trauma**
– **...**

Structural changes like
– biochemical alterations of muscle tissue
– fat infiltration after trauma
– atrophy reflected by reduced CSA
– fibre transformation from type I to II
– ...

Functional changes like
– lower activity of the deep cervical muscles
– higher activity of the superficial cervical muscles
– lower directional specificity
– higher coactivation
– delayed onset and offset (relaxation) of muscle activation
– ...

Outcomes
Less strength, limited endurance, reduced head-eye coordination, altered coordination and proprioception, ...

Fig. 48. Functional and structural changes in muscles related to pain (adapted from Falla and Farina 2007)

The alterations in motor control associated with pain can be considered a compensatory mechanism to maintain similar motor output in painful and non-painful conditions [57]. Overload and trauma are well-recognized release mechanisms for the initiation of pain and motor dysfunction for example after a whiplash injury [52, 55]. Disuse is a further obvious although often neglected cause and/or maintaining factor of functional and structural changes. It represents a starting point for active rehabilitation programs for patients with neck pain.

5.2 EFFICACY OF EXERCISE FOR PATIENTS WITH NECK PAIN

Patients with traumatic onset of neck pain have shown significantly increased prevalence of combined rotational and translational hypermobility in the middle cervical spine segments (C3-4 to C5-6) compared to women with insidious onset of neck pain [263]. The increased tension on different spinal structures which might result from this hypermobility is considered a major source of pain [246]. Valid and reliable clinical tests for the diagnosis of minor clinical instability or hypermobility are lacking [264, 265] although there is a consensus on typical clinical findings [266].

One essential part of the treatment of this hypermobility is active exercise. Moderate evidence for its efficacy exists when exercises are performed alone and strong evidence when they are combined with mobilization or manipulation for subacute and chronic mechanical neck disorders with or without headache in the short and long term for pain reduction, improved function, and they have a high global perceived effect [18]. An isometric extension with increasing resistance in the neutral position of the head will recruit the deep and superficial extensors as observed with EMG [99, 100] and ultrasonography which showed increasing thickness of multifidus during extension from 0 to 50% MVC [182]. The specific dysfunctions of cervical muscles observed in various studies suggest that appropriate specific exercises with a certain dosage are necessary for the treatment of muscle dysfunction and neck pain. Generally, exercises are divided into low- and high-load exercises.

Low-load exercises mainly aim at functional adaptation and motor control strategies and improve activation and coordination of selected muscles such as the deep cervical flexors and extensors. High-load exercises on the contrary aim at morphological adaptations and to ameliorate endurance and strength of selected muscles and movements and are usually introduced later in the rehabilitation program [267].

A classical low load exercise is craniocervical flexion which has largely been investigated as test and exercise for patients with neck pain resulting in specific activation of the deep cervical flexors [268]. It aims successfully to re-establish a normal activation pattern of superficial and deep cervical flexor muscles [22, 23] and to reduce pain [24]. Furthermore, it induces immediate local hypoalgesia after a single training session (21% reduction of PPT compared to 7.3% after cervical flexion exercise), but no change of local thermal pain threshold and no effect on the sympathetic nervous system, pain at a location distant from the cervical spine and neck pain at rest [25]. These low intensity exercises are believed to be indicated especially in the early phase of rehabilitation in order to activate selectively the inhibited deep muscles [27].

An isometric cervical flexion endurance exercise (lifting and holding the head 1 cm from the treatment table) increases the load and activates more the lower cervical flexors [76, 78] with similar activation of the craniocervical flexors to the craniocervical flexion exercise, but with more activity in the sternocleidomastoid, the anterior scalene, and the suprahyoid muscles [268]. It seems important to adapt the treatment to the individual dysfunction of each patient because even treatment of the superficial sternocleidomastoid muscle can be effective for pain reduction in the case of an asymmetry for example [269].

High load exercises alleviate pain and improve several functional parameters [270-272] like endurance [273] and strength [16, 274]. Twelve weeks of strength resistance exercises for example with maximal resistance to the head (75% and 100% of 3x10 RM) increased the head-extension strength by 34%. Namely the primary extensors (splenius capitis, semispinalis capitis and semispinalis cervicis with multifidus) increased their strength, while the other extensors decreased their activity in the neck extension group reflecting the increased strength of the former muscles as measured by muscle functional MRI [137]. High load exercises however risk to increase pain in the early phase of rehabilitation [42]. Improvements in muscle function by exercise seem to be task specific, i.e. specific to the exercise [275]. Strength in cervical flexion for example can be increased by cervical flexion endurance-strength training but not by the low-load exercise of craniocervical flexion [273]. Specific exercises consequently seem necessary in order to increase the reduced activity of the deep cervical extensors in patients with neck pain. One study investigated with mfMRI the activation of the extensor muscles in healthy subjects during isometric extension at 20% MVC and showed greater activity with the spine in 15° of craniocervical extension for semispinalis capitis at levels C2-3 and C5-6 and in multifidus with semispinalis cervicis at level C7-T1 compared to the exercise with the spine in craniocervical neutral position [245]. Using the same exercise patients with neck pain showed reduced activation of multifidus with semispinalis cervicis in the craniocervical neutral position at levels C5-6 and C7-T1 compared to healthy controls, but not at level C2-3 [98]. At level C7-T1 but not C2-3 this lower activation of the deep cervical extensors occurred also in healthy subjects with experimental pain in the upper trapezius [124]. The exercise shown in study 4 of this thesis is the first one showing increased activation of semispinalis cervicis at level C3 in patients with chronic neck pain relative to the superficial splenius capitis. This was achieved by asking the patient to push against a manual resistance applied at the vertebral arch of C2. With this exercise the way is open now to assess the efficacy of the emphasized activation of semispinalis cervicis in a large RCT on patients with chronic neck pain.

5.3 IMPLICATIONS FOR REHABILITATION

These findings are highly relevant for patients with neck pain because the activity of their deep semispinalis cervicis muscle which is lower compared to healthy controls can be increased relative to the superficial splenius capitis muscle by a specific exercise.

The independent neural input to fascicles of semispinalis cervicis at spinal levels C2 and C5 found in study one might allow to selectively activate the deep extensor(s) at the most symptomatic spinal level respectively the one with major dysfunction(s) using specific exercises. Further research however is necessary in this regard because clinical detection of the most affected segments is still questioned [276, 277]. Studies 2 and 3 have shown a lower activation and lower directional specificity of semispinalis cervicis at different spinal levels in patients with neck pain compared to healthy controls. This might suggest specific exercises for activation of this muscle – and probably also for the other deep extensor multifidus - as part of the rehabilitation of patients with neck pain.

Contrary to study 2 and 3, O'Leary et al. [98] did not find lower activity of semispinalis cervicis at level C2-3 in patients with chronic neck pain, but only at levels C5-6 and C7-T1 and only with the head in craniocervical neutral position. This might partially be explained by the functional redundancy of the neck muscles which allows the nervous system to use different muscles for a given task [100]. The variability of individual EMG findings reflected in the standard deviations of the presented studies might equally be explained by this functional redundancy of the neck muscles. At higher loads however muscles that contribute specifically to generate the required load in a desired direction are recruited [100] suggesting that activation of selected cervical extensors might require higher resistance than the 15 and 30N used in this thesis or the 20% MVC used by O'Leary et al. [98]. Indeed, the exercise in study 4 showing increased activation of semispinalis cervicis relative to splenius capitis was done with the patient's maximum force. Also a strength training with 80% MVC in healthy subjects over 12 weeks results in increased cross-sectional area of semispinalis cervicis, semispinalis capitis, and splenius capitis [278] and a decreased use of these muscles reflecting increased force as measured with functional MRI [137]. However, these high-load exercises cannot be used in the early stage of rehabilitation [27].

The resistance in study 4 was neither standardized nor measured in order to reflect the clinical use of the exercise intensity which is adapted to each individual patient's ability to bear stress. It was at the individual painless maximum intensity which is probably the nearest point to the training threshold, i.e. the intensity where morphological and physiological adaptations of the muscle following a stimulus (exercise) start [279]. The simplicity of the exercise facilitates its use as a self-exercise by putting a towel or belt around the neck and pulling it ventrally while pushing backwards into extension with the neck. Based on the available evidence it can therefore be recommended to activate the deep cervical extensors by manual resistances applied at the vertebral arch at possibly the maximum voluntary contraction force without provoking any immediate or delayed pain.

5.4 METHODOLOGICAL CONSIDERATIONS

Some limitations prevent a rapid generalization of these results. The small sample size in the studies might have led to "false positive" results equivalent to a type I error. This flaw could have been counteracted by increasing the number of participants in the studies. Ethical reasons however, due to the invasive nature of the EMG procedure limited the number of participants which is in line with similar studies in the literature.

Furthermore, a selection bias may have occurred during the recruitment process by the announcement of needle insertion. Subjects with fear of pain might have even not considered participating in the studies due to the supposed "threat" of needle insertion. Fear of pain is believed to limit force for example in patients with neck pain following a whiplash injury [72] and consequently it might be that only "fearless" subjects have volunteered for this project. This flaw cannot be overcome by increasing the number of participants. New non-invasive technology like mfMRI [98] and tissue velocity ultrasound imaging [138] might be able to avoid this selection bias and the recruitment limitation due to needle insertion although it is not clear whether these measurements are equivalent to EMG. A selection bias may have occurred also by using some patients in more than one experiment due to recruitment difficulties (see page 27).

A further limitation is the motor task which is not reflecting daily activity but was selected for reasons of standardization. It might be questionable whether the results from these exercises are transferable to other activities.

Other statistical tests than the ANOVA might have been used to analyse the data as their normality has been checked only by the Kolmogorov-Smirnov test. Due to the small sample size non-parametric tests might have an additional option for data analysis.

Moreover, the sequence of exercises in study 4 has not been randomized. This might have biased the results due to a possible learning effect at the second exercise (resistance at C2) and a possible fatigue effect at the third exercise (resistance at C5). The difference betrween the first and second exercise however was big for which reason we do not assume a learning effect. In addition patients did not report subjective fatigue during or after the third exercise.

It is still unclear whether manual resistance at single spinal levels can activate the deep extensors at selected levels like the most painful one. This thesis showed that reduced EMG activity and directional specificity is a generalized phenomenon at several spinal levels. This however is based on the mean values of all subjects. Future research might investigate whether EMG activity in patients with neck pain is lower at the most symptomatic level compared to other spinal levels and whether it can selectively be increased at these levels. The most painful segment however can only be identified in a valid way by invasive techniques like selective nerve blocks of the zygapophyseal joints or discography in highly specialized pain clinics [2]. After such invasive diagnostic procedures it is uncertain whether these patients would volunteer for further needle insertions in an experiment what represents also an ethical question. Such an investigation would be further complicated by the necessary amount of wires inserted into the muscle fibres which would make it difficult to apply the resistance at the vertebral arch without provoking EMG artefacts.

5.5 FUTURE RESEARCH

The ultimate goal of the research on the deep cervical extensors is to find out if a specific exercise like the one from study 4 successfully reduces the patient's neck pain and dysfunction. This raises the questions whether an exercise stimulating the deep extensors more than the superficial ones is more effective compared to a general exercise and whether it is necessary to apply the exercise in the segment with most pain. Analogous to the previously described research on the cervical flexors it might be probable that an exercise emphasizing the deep cervical extensors would be most effective. In order to reduce neck pain, mobilization [280, 281] and manipulation [11, 282, 283] do not have to be applied to the most painful cervical segment, but can even be performed in the upper thoracic spine. It is believed, that exercises should be directed to specific spinal levels in order to improve the function [27] but no research regarding this question exists up to now. Using RCTs these questions could be answered even with a high number of participants without using high technology like iEMG. The lack of internal validity would be counterbalanced by a gain in external validity.

Chapter 6.

General conclusions

This thesis investigated the deep cervical extensor semispinalis cervicis in healthy volunteers and patients with chronic neck pain. The anatomical characteristics of this muscle allow movement control and stabilization of single cervical segments caudal to C2 together with other muscles of the cervical spine. Study 1 confirmed this possibility by revealing independent synaptic input to different fascicles of semispinalis cervicis at levels C2 and C5. The significance of semispinalis cervicis was shown in study 2 by lower EMG activity and directional specificity at level C3 in patients with chronic neck pain compared to healthy controls. This phenomenon was also observed at the levels C2 and C5 in study 3. At these levels PPT over the zygapophyseal joints was lower in the patients compared to healthy controls. In both groups PPT at C2 was lower compared to C5 indicating a generally higher tissue sensitivity to pressure at level C2. Taking both groups together this tissue sensitivity correlated significantly, albeit weakly, to EMG activity and directional specificity at levels C2 and C5 indicating a small influence of tissue sensitivity on the activation of the semispinalis cervicis muscle. Other factors besides pain might influence EMG activity and directional specificity such as disuse and fear of pain.

The results of this thesis support the importance of specific exercise in the treatment of patients with chronic neck pain. An appropriate exercise for activation of semispinalis cervicis relative to the superficial splenius capitis was investigated in study 4. This exercise might be important for restoring normal muscle function in patients with chronic neck pain. Further research has to assess this potential effect.

Appendixes

APPENDIX 1: COMMON METHODS

The following table gives an overview on the common methods used in this thesis.

Section	Study 1	Study 2	Study 3	Study 4
Title	Recruitment of motor units in two fascicles of the semispinalis cervicis muscle	Chronic trauma-induced neck pain impairs the neural control of the deep semispinalis cervicis muscle	Localized pain sensitivity is associated with reduced activation of the semispinalis cervicis muscle in patients with neck pain	Localised resistance selectively activates the semispinalis cervicis muscle in patients with neck pain
Main research question	Is there an independent synaptic input to different fascicles of semispinalis cervicis at C2 and C5 level?	Is the EMG activity of semispinalis cervicis different between patients and controls?	Is the activity of semispinalis cervicis related to pressure pain sensitivity at levels C2 and C5?	Can a specific exercise selectively increase the activation of semispinalis cervicis compared to a superficial extensor?

Table 2: Overview of the methods from studies 1 to 4 (continuation see next page)

Section	Study 1	Study 2	Study 3	Study 4
Study design	Cross-sectional	idem	idem	Repeated measures
Subject inclusion criteria	Age between 18 and 45 years, no neck pain, no history of neck surgery or neurological disorders	Patients: age 18 – 45 yr pain duration > 3 months pain > 3 VAS Controls: no neck pain, no history of neck surgery or neurological disorders		
Exclusion criteria	Complaints of neurological signs, neurological signs on clinical assessment, cervical spine surgery, and/or neck pain			
Subjects	1st experiment: 7 women (age, mean ± SD: 24.1 ± 2.9 yr) and 8 men (age: 24.2 ± 1.9 yr) 2nd experiment: 8 healthy women (age, mean, SD: 26.0 ± 2.7 yr)	10 women with neck pain (> 6 months; 30.4 ± 7.0 yr) and 10 healthy women (26.8 ± 5.9 yr)	10 women with neck pain (> 6 months; 34 ± 8.8 yr) and 9 healthy women (27 ± 4.1 yr)	10 women with neck pain (> 6 months; 31.9 ± 7.7 yr)

Continuation of table 2: Overview of the methods from studies 1 to 4 (continuation see next page)

Section	Study 1	Study 2	Study 3	Study 4
Cause of neck pain	no pain	all trauma	9 trauma, 1 stress	all trauma
Average pain intensity (VAS) (mean ± SD)	no pain	5.8 ± 1.6	6.1 ± 2.0	6.1 ± 1.5
Neck Disability Index (NDI) (mean ± SD)	no disability	21.2 ± 5.7	19.6 ± 7.5	23 ± 4.8
Target muscles	Semispinalis cervicis	Semispinalis cervicis	Semispinalis cervicis	Semispinalis cervicis and splenius capitis
EMG	1st experiment: single MU analysis 2nd experiment: interference EMG	interference EMG	interference EMG	interference EMG
Location of wire insertion	C2 and C5	C3	C2 and C5	C3
Side of insertion	Right side	Patients: most painful side (8 right), controls right side	Patients: most painful side (8 right), controls right side	Most painful side (8 right),

Continuation of table 2: Overview of the methods from studies 1 to 4 (continuation see next page)

Section	Study 1	Study 2	Study 3	Study 4
Performed test movement	Isometric extension 1st experiment: 3 MVC without wires sustained (120 s) and ramped (3s) 2nd experiment: 2 MVC and 5 s ramped	2 MVC in extension circular contractions 0-360° at 15 and 30N over 12 s each	circular contractions 0-360° at 15 and 30N over 12 s each	Isometric extension against manual resistances at occiput and at vertebral arches of C2 and C5
Outcome measure	1st experiment: MVC Number of MU Discharge rate Coefficient of variation of ISI Short-term synchronization (CIS) Coherence analysis recruitment threshold 2nd experiment: MVC and amplitude of interference EMG	MVC: highest peak value of 2 MVCs of 5 s each Amplitude of interference EMG Vector length of the directional activation curve with coefficient of force	Amplitude of interference EMG Vector length of the directional activation curve PPT	Amplitude of interference EMG (average rectified value)

Continuation of table 2: Overview of the methods from studies 1 to 4. Further details are in chapter 3

APPENDIX 2: OVERVIEW OF THE RESULTS

The following table gives an overview on the results.

Table 3. Overview of the results

	General result	Detailed result
Study 1	There is an independent synaptic input to fascicles of semispinalis cervicis at levels C2 and C5.	*1ˢᵗ experiment:* N° of MUs: C2 18 and C5 98 Discharge rate: equal between C2 and C5 but higher at 20% MVC compared to 5% and 10% MVC Coefficient of variation ISI: equal between both levels and across all 3 force levels Short-term synchronization and coherence in the frequency: similar and higher within levels than between Recruitment threshold lower at C5 than at C2 *2ⁿᵈ experiment:* higher amplitude with increasing force and higher amplitude at C5 than at C2
Study 2	EMG activity is reduced in patients compared to controls.	Extension strength, mean EMG activity and directional specificity were lower for patients than for controls at level C3 while the coefficient of variation of force was higher in patients.
Study 3	Lower PPT is correlated to lower EMG activity in patients with neck pain at levels C2 and C5.	PPT was lower in patients and differed between C2 and C5 and was correlated to EMG activity and directional specificity at both which showed no difference between spinal and force levels.
Study 4	A specific exercise can increase activity of the semispinalis cervicis relative to splenius capitis	Resistance applied at C2 increased the activity of semispinalis cervicis relative to splenius capitis as measured at level C3 compared to resistances applied at the occiput and at C5 level.

References

1.   Niemeläinen R, Videman T, Battié MC. Prevalence and characteristics of upper or mid-back pain in Finnish men. Spine 2006;31(16):1846-9.

2.   Bogduk N, McGuirk B. Management of acute and chronic neck pain, An evidence-based approach. Edinburgh ... Elsevier; 2006.

3.   Freburger JK, Carey TS, Holmes GM. Management of back and neck pain: who seeks care from physical therapists? Physical Therapy 2005;85(9):872-68.

4.   Chow RT, Heller GZ, Barnsley L. The effect of 300 mW, 830 nm laser on chronic neck pain: a double-blind, randomized, placebo-controlled study. Pain 2006;124(1-2):201-10.

5.   Gustavsson C, Denison E, von Koch L. Self-management of persistent neck pain: a randomized controlled trial of a multi-component group intervention in primary health care. European Journal of Pain 2010;14(6):630.e1-.e11.

6.   Sherman KJ, Cherkin DC, Hawkes RJ, Miglioretti DL, Deyo RA. Randomized trial of therapeutic massage for chronic neck pain. Clinical Journal of Pain 2009;25(3):233-8.

7.   Kanlayanaphotporn R, Chiradejnant A, Vachalathiti R. The immediate effects of mobilization technique on pain and range of motion in patients presenting with unilateral neck pain: A randomized controlled trial. Archives of Physical Medicine and Rehabilitation 2009;90:187-92.

8.   Schomacher J. The Effect of an Analgesic Mobilization Technique when Applied at Symptomatic or Asymptomatic Levels of the Cervical Spine in Subjects with Neck Pain: A Randomized Controlled Trial. Journal of Manual & Manipulative Therapy 2009;17(2):101-8.

9.   Lau HM, Wing Chiu TT, Lam TH. The effectiveness of thoracic manipulation on patients with chronic mechanical neck pain - a randomized controlled trial. Manual Therapy 2011;16(2):141-7.

10.   Krauss J, Creighton D, Ely JD, Podlewska-Ely J. The immediate effects of upper thoracic translatoric spinal manipulation on cervical pain and range of motion: A randomized clinical trial. The Journal of Manual & Manipulative Therapy 2008;16(2):93-9.

11.   Cleland JA, Childs JD, McRae M, Palmer JA, Stowell T. Immediate effects of thoracic manipulation in patients with neck pain: a randomized clinical trial. Manual Therapy 2005;10:127-35.

12.   Cleland JA, Glynn P, Whitman JM, Eberhart SL, MacDonald C, Childs JD. Short-term effects of thrust versus nonthrust mobilization/manipulation directed at the throacic spine in patients with neck pain: a randomized clinical trial. Physical Therapy 2007;87(4):431-40.

13.   Haraldsson BG, Gross AR, Myers CD, Ezzo JM, Morien A, Goldsmith C et al. Massage for mechanical neck disorders (Review). Cochrane Database of Systematic Reviews 2006(3):1-61.

14.   Gross A, Miller J, D'Sylva J, Burnie SJ, Goldsmith CH, Graham N et al. Manipulation or mobilisation for neck pain: A Corane Review. Manual Therapy 2010;15(4):315-33.

15.   Stewart MJ, Maher CG, Refshauge KM, Herbert RD, Bogduk N, Nicholas M. Randomized controlled trial of exercise for chronic whiplash-associated disorders. Pain 2007;120(1-2):59-68.

16.   Ylinen J, Takala E-P, Nykänen M, Häkkinen AH, Mälkiä E, Pohjolainen T et al. Active neck muscle training in the treatment of chronic neck pain in women. JAMA (The journal of the American Medical Association) 2003;289(19):2509-16.

17.   Jull G, Falla D, Treleaven J, Hodges PW, Vicenzino B. Retraining cervical joint position sense: the effect of two exercise regimes. Journal of Orthopaedic Research 2007;25:404-12.

18.   Kay TM, Gross A, Goldsmith C, Santaguida PL, Hoving JL, Bronfort G et al. Exercise for mechanical neck disorders. Cochrane Database of Systematic Reviews 2005(3. Art. No.: CD004250).

19.   Ylinen J. Physical exercises and functional rehabilitation for the management of chronic neck pain. Europa Medicophysica 2007;43:119-32.

20.   Falla D, Jull G, Hodges PW. Patients with neck pain demonstrate reduced electromyographic activity of the deep cervical flexor muscles during performance of the craniocervical flexion test. Spine 2004;29(19):2108-14.

21.   Falla D, Bilenkij G, Jull G. Patients with chronic neck pain demonstrate altered patterns of muscle activation during performance of a functional upper limb task. Spine 2004;29(13):1436-40.

22.   Jull G, Falla D, Treleaven J, Sterling M, O'Leary S. A therapeutic exercise approach for cervical disorders. In: Boyling JD, Jull G, editors. Grieve's modern manual therapy: the vertebral column. 3rd ed. Edinburgh: Elsevier; 2004.

23.   Sterling M, Jull G, Wright A. Cervical mobilisation: concurrent effects on pain, sympathetic nervous system activity and motor activity. Manual Therapy 2001;6(^2):72-81.

24.   Jull G, Trott P, Potter H, Zito G, Niere KR, Shirley D et al. A randomized controlled trial of exercise and manipulative therapy for cervicogenic headache. Spine 2002;27:1835-43.

25.   O'Leary S, Falla D, Hodges PW, Jull G, Vicenzino B. Specific therapeutic exercise of the neck induces immediate local hypoalgesia. The Journal of Pain 2007;8(11):832-9.

26.   Falla D, O'Leary SP, Farina D, Jull G. The change in deep cervical flexor activity after training is associated with the degree of pain reduction in patients with chronic neck pain. Clinical Journal of Pain 2011;28(7):628-34.

27.   O'Leary S, Falla D, Elliott JM, Jull G. Muscle dysfunction in cervical spine pain: implications for assessment and management. Journal of Orthopaedic & Sports Physical Therapy 2009;39(5):324-33.

28.   Fejer R, Kyvik KO, Hartvigsen J. The prevalence of neck pain in the world population: a systematic critical review of the literature. European Spine Journal 2006;15:834-48.

29.   Chiu TT, Leung AS. Neck pain in Hong Kong, a telephone survey on prevalence, consequences, and risk groups. Spine 2006;31(16):E540-E4.
30.   Côté P, Cassidy D, Caroll L, Kristman V. The annual incidence and course of neck pain in the general population: a population-based cohort study. Pain 2004;112:267-73.
31.   Côté P, Cassidy D, Caroll L. The Saskatchewan health and back pain survey, the prevalence of neck pain and related disability in Saskatchewan adults. Spine 1998;23(15):1689-98.
32.   Guez M, Hildingsson C, Nilsson M, Toolanen G. The prevalence of neck pain, A population-based study from northern Sweden. Acta orthopaedica Scandinavica 2002;73(4):455-9.
33.   Bovim G, Schrader H, Sand T. Neck pain in the general population. Spine 1994;19(12):1307-9.
34.   Croft PR, Lewis M, Papageorgiou AC, Thomas E, Jason MIV, Macfarlane GJ et al. Risk factors for neck pain: a longitudinal study in the general population. Pain 2001;93:317-25.
35.   Picavet HSJ, Schouten JSAG. Musculoskeletal pain in the Netherlands: prevalences, consequences and risk groups, the DMC3-study. Pain 2003;102:167-78.
36.   Ylinen J, Kautiainen H, Wirén K, Häkkinen AH. Stretching exercises vs manual therapy in treatment of chronic neck pain: a randomized, controlled cross-over trial. Journal of Rehabilitation Medicine 2007;39:126-32.
37.   Kjellman G, Öberg B, Hensing G, Alexanderson K. A 12-year follow-up of subjects initially sicklisted with neck/shoulder or low back diagnoses. Physiotherapy Research International 2001;6(1):52-63.
38.   Holmberg SAC, Thelin AG. Primary care consultation, hospital admission, sick leave and disability pension owing to neck and low back pain: a 12-year prospective cohort study in a rural population. BMC Musculoskeletal Disorders 2006;7(66).
39.   Carroll LJ, Haldeman S, Carragee EJ, Nordin M, Guzman J. Course and prognostic factors for neck pain in the general population, Results of the Bone and Joint Decade 2000-2010 task Force on Neck Pain and Its Associated Disorders. Journal of Manipulative and Physiological Therapeutics 2009;32:S87-S96.
40.   Korthals de Bos IBC, Hoving JL, van Tulder MW, Tutten Van Molken MPMH, Ader HJ, de Vet HCW et al. Cost effectiveness of physiotherapy, manual therapy, and general practitioner care for neck pain: economic evaluation alongside a randomised controlled trial. Britisch Medical Journal 2003;236(7395):911 - 4B.
41.   Borghouts JAJ, Koes BW, Vondeling H, Bouter LM. Cost-of-illness of neck pain in the Netherlands in 1996. Pain 1999;80:629-236.
42.   Jull G, Sterling M, Falla D, Treleaven J, O'Leary S. Whiplash, Headache, and Neck Pain: Research-Based Directions for Physical Therapies: Research-based directions for physical therapies. Edinburgh ... Churchill Livingstone (Elsevier); 2008.
43.   Hviid Andersen J, Kaergaard A, Frost P, Frolund Thomsen J, Peter Bonde J, Fallentin N et al. Physical, psychosocial, and individual risk factors for

neck/shoulder pain with pressure tenderness in the muscles among workers performing monotonous, repetitive work. Spine 2002;27(6):660-7.

44. Manchikanti L, Dunbar EE, Wargo BW, Shah RV, Derby R, Cohen SP. Systematic review of cervical discography as a diagnostic test for chronic spinal pain. Pain Physician 2009;12:305-21.

45. Slipman CW, Plastaras C, Patel R, Isaac Z, Chow D, Garavan C et al. Provocative cervical discography symptom mapping. The Spine Journal 2005;5:381-8.

46. Aprill C, Bogduk N. The prevalence of cervical zygapophyseal joint pain, A First Approximation. Spine 1992;17(7):744-7.

47. Lord S, Barnsley L, Wallis BJ, Bogduk N. Chronic cervical zygapophysial joint pain after whiplash. Spine 1996;21(15):1737-45.

48. Bogduk N, Marsland A. The cervical zygapophysial joints as a source of neck pain. Spine 1988;13(6):610-7.

49. Barnsley L, Lord SM, Wallis BJ, Bogduk N. The prevalence of chronic cervical zygapophysial joint pain after whiplash. Spine 1995;20(1):20-6.

50. Aprill C, Dwyer A, Bogduk N. Cervical zygapophyseal joint pain patterns II: a clinical evaluation. Spine 1990;15(6):458-61.

51. Dwyer A, Aprill C, Bogduk N. Cervical zygapophyseal joint pain patterns I: a study in normal volunteers. Spine 1990;15(6):453-7.

52. Bogduk N, Yoganandan N. Biomechanics of the cervical spine. Part 3: minor injuries. Clinical Biomechanics 2001;16:267-75.

53. Wainner RS, Fritz JM, Irrgang JJ, Boninger ML, Delitto A, Allison S. The Reliability and diagnostic accuracy of clinical examination and patient self-report measures for cervical radiculopathy. Spine 2003;28(1):52-62.

54. Panjabi MM. The stabilizing system of the spine. Part II. Neutral zone and instability hypothesis. Journal of spinal disorders & techniques 1992;5:390-7.

55. Pearson AM, Ivanicic PC, Ito S, Panjabi MM. Facet joint kinematics and injury mechanisms during simulated whiplash. Spine 2004;29(4):390-7.

56. Wen N, Lavaste F, Santin JJ, Lassau JP. Three-dimensional biomechanical properties of the human cervical spine in vitro, II. Analysis of instability after ligamentous injuries. European Spine Journal 1993;2:12-5.

57. Falla D, Farina D. Neuromuscular adaptation in experimental and clinical neck pain. Journal of Electromyography and Kinesiology 2008;18:255-61.

58. Falla D, Farina D, Graven-Nielsen T. Experimental muscle pain results in reorganization of coordination among trapezius muscle subdivisions during repetitive shoulder flexion. Experimental Brain Research 2006;178(3):385-93.

59. Lucas KR, Plolus BI, Rich PA. Latent myofascial trigger points: their effects on muscle activation and movement efficiency. Journal of Bodywork and Movement Therapies 2004;8:160-6.

60. Jones MA, Rivett DA. Clinical reasoning for manual therapists. Edinburgh ... Butterworth Heinemann; 2004.

61. Jull G, Amiri M, Bullock-Saxton J, Darnell R, Lander C. Cervical musculoskeletal impairment in frequent intermittent headache. Part 1: Subjects with single headaches. Cephalgia 2007;27:793-802.

62. Masi AT, Nannon JC. Human resting muscle tone (HRMT): narrative introduction and modern concepts. Journal of bodywork and movement therapies 2008;12(4):320-32.
63. Laube W, Müller K. Muskeltonus als biophysikalische und neurophysiologische Zustandsgröße – Passiver Muskeltonus. Manuelle Therapie. Manuelle Therapie 2002;6(1):21-30.
64. Keshner EA. Head-trunk coordination during linear anterior-posterior translations. Journal of Neurophysiology 2003;89:1891-901.
65. Danna-Dos-Santos A, Degani AM, Latash ML. Anticipatory control of head posture. Clinical Neurophysiology 2007;118:1802-14.
66. Panjabi MM, Cholewicki J, Nibu K, Grauer J, Babat LB, Dvorak J. Critical load of the human cervical spine: an in vitro experimental study. Clinical Biomechanics 1998;13(1):11-7.
67. Bexander CSM, Mellor R, Hodges PW. Effect of gaze direction on neck muscle activity during cervical rotation. Experimental Brain Research 2005;167:422-32.
68. Kristjansson E, Treleaven J. Sensorimotor function and dizziness in neck pain: implications for assessment and management. Journal of Orthopaedic & Sports Physical Therapy 2009;39(5):364-77.
69. Armstrong B, McNair P, Taylor D. Head and neck position sense. Sports Medicine 2008;38(2):101-17.
70. Jull GA. Considerations in the physical rehabilitation of patients with whiplash-associated disorders. Spine 2011;36(25 Suppl):S286-S91.
71. Lindstroem R, Falla D. Current pain and fear of pain contribute to reduced maximum voluntary contraction of neck muscles in patients with chronic neck pain. Archives of Physical Medicine and Rehabilitation 2012.
72. Prushansky T, Gepstein R, Gordon C, Dvir Z. Cervical muscles weakness in chronic whiplash patients. Clinical Biomechanics 2005;20:794-8.
73. Lindstrøm R, Schomacher J, Farina D, Rechter L, Falla D. Association between neck muscle coactivation, pain, and strength in women with neck pain. Manual Therapy 2011;16(1):80-6.
74. Ylinen J, Salo PK, Nykänen M, Kautiainen H, Häkkinen AH. Decreased isometric neck strength in women with chronic neck pain and the repeatability of neck strength measurements. Archives of Physical Medicine and Rehabilitation 2004;85:1303-8.
75. Ylinen J, Takala E-P, Kautiainen H, Nykänen M, Häkkinen AH, Pohjolainen T et al. Association of neck pain, disability and neck pain during maximal effort with neck muscle strength and range of movement in women with chronic non-specific neck pain. European Journal of Pain 2004;8:473-8.
76. Grimmer KA. Measuring the endurance capacity of the cervical short flexor muscle group. Australian Journal of Physiotherapy 1994;40(4):251-4.
77. Piper A. Vergleich der Ausdauerleistungsfähigkeit der vorwiegend tiefen Flexoren der Halswirbelsäule (HWS) zwischen Gesunden und Probanden mit HWS-Schmerz. Manuelle Therapie 2009;13(5).

78.   Cagnie B, Dickx N, Peeters I, Tuytens J, Achten E, Cambier D et al. The use of functional MRI to evaluate cervical flexor activity during different cervical flexion exercises. Journal of Applied Physiology 2008;104:230-5.

79.   de Koning CHP, van den Heuvel SP, Staal JB, Smits-Engelsman BC, Hendriks EJ. Clinimetric evaluation of methods to measure muscle functioning in patients with non-specific neck pain: a systematic review. BMC Musculoskeletal Disorders 2008;9.

80.   Jull G, Kristjansson E, Dall'Alba P. Impairment in the cervical flexors: a comparison of whiplash and insidious onset neck pain patients. Manual Therapy 2004;9:89-94.

81.   Biering-Sørensen F. Physical measurements as risk indicators for low-back trouble over a one-year period. Spine 1984;9(2):106-19.

82.   Lee H, Nicholson LL, Adams RD. Neck muscle endurance, self-report, and range of motion data from subjects with treated and untreated neck pain. Journal of Manipulative and Physiological Therapeutics 2005;28:25-32.

83.   Edmonston SJ, Björnsdóttir G, Pálsson T, Solgård H, Ussing K, Allison G. Endurance and fatigue characteristics of the neck flexor and extensor muscles during isometric tests in patients with postural neck pain. Manual Therapy 2011;16:332-8.

84.   Falla D, Rainoldi A, Merletti R, Jull G. Myoelectric manifestations of sternocleidomastoid and anterior scalene muscle fatigue in chronic neck pain patients. Clinical Neurophysiology 2003;114:488-95.

85.   Falla D, Jull G, Rainoldi A, Merletti R. Neck flexor muscle fatigue is side specific in patients with unilateral neck pain. European Journal of Pain 2004;8(1):71-7.

86.   Falla D, Jull G, Dall'Alba P, Rainoldi A, Merletti R. An electromyographic analysis of the deep cervical flexor muscles in performance of craniocervical flexion. Physical Therapy 2003;83(10):899-906.

87.   Falla D, Jull G, O'Leary S, Dall'Alba P. Further evaluation of an EMG technique for assessment of the deep cervical flexor muscles. Journal of Elektromyography and Kinesiology 2006;16:621-8.

88.   Sterling M, Jull G, Vicenzino B, Kenardy J, Darnell R. Development of motor system dysfunction following whiplash injury. Pain 2003;103:65-73.

89.   O'Leary SP, Falla D, Jull G. The relationship between superficial muscle activity during the cranio-cervical flexion test and clinical features in patients with chronic neck pain. Manual Therapy 2011;16:452-5.

90.   Falla D, Jull G, Hodges PW. Feedforward activity of the cervical flexor muscles during voluntary arm movements is delayed in chronic neck pain. Experimental Brain Research 2004;157:43-8.

91.   Falla D, O'Leary S, Farina D, Jull G. Association between intensity of pain and impairment in onset and activation of the deep cervical flexors in patients with persistent neck pain. Clinical Journal of Pain 2011;27:309-14.

92.   Falla D, Lindstrøm R, Rechter L, Farina D. Effect of pain on modulation in discharge rate of sternocleidomastoid motor units with force direction. Clinical Neurophysiology 2010;121(5):744-53.

93.   Johnston V, Jull G, Souvlis T, Jimmieson N. Neck movement and muscle activity characteristics in female office workers with neck pain. Spine 2008;33(5):555-63.

94.   O'Sullivan PB, Beales DJ. Diagnosis and classification of pelvic girdle pain disorders – Part 1: A mechanism based approach within a biopsychosocial framework. Manual Therapy 2007;12:86-97.

95.   O'Sullivan P. Diagnosis and classification of chronic low back pain disorders: Maladaptive Movement and motor control impairments as underlying mechanism. Manual Therapy 2005;10(4):242-55.

96.   Szeto GPY, Straker LM, O'Sullivan PB. A comparison of symptomatic and asymptomatic office workers performing monotonous keyboard work – 1: Neck and shoulder muscle recruitment patterns. Manual Therapy 2005;10:270-80.

97.   Kumar S, Narayan Y, Prasad N, Shuaib A, Siddiqui ZA. Cervical electromyogram profile differences between patients of neck pain and control. Spine 2007;32(8):E246-E53.

98.   O'Leary S, Cagnie B, Reeve A, Jull G, Elliott JM. Is there altered activity of the extensor muscles in chronic mechanical neck pain? A functional magnetic resonance imaging study. Archives of Physical Medicine and Rehabilitation 2011;92:929-34.

99.   Mayoux-Benhamou MA, Revel M, Vallee C. Selective electromyography of dorsal neck muscles in humans. Experimental Brain Research 1997;113:353-60.

100.   Blouin J-S, Siegmund GP, Carpenter MG, Inglis JT. Neural control of superficial and deep neck muscles in humans. Journal of Neurophysiology 2007;98:920-8.

101.   Valkeinen H, Ylinen J, Mälkiä E, Markku, Häkkinen K. Maximal force, force/time and activation/coactivation characteristics of the neck muscles in extension and flexion in healthy men and women at different ages. European Journal of Applied Physiology 2002;88:247-54.

102.   Enoka RM. Neural adaptations with chronic physical activity. Journal of Biomechanics 1997;30(5):447-55.

103.   Cheng C-H, Lin K-H, Wang J-L. Co-contraction of cervical muscles during sagittal and coronal neck motions at different movement speeds. European Journal of Applied Physiology 2008;103:647-54.

104.   Miljkovic-Gacic I, Wang W, Kammerer CM, Gordon CL, Bunker CH, Kuller LH et al. Fat infiltration in muscle: new evidence for familial clustering and associations with diabetes. Obesity (Silver Spring) 2008;16(8):1854-60.

105.   Melis B, DeFranco MJ, Chuinard C, Walch G. Natural history of fatty infiltration and atrophy of the supraspinatus muscle in rotator cuff tears. Clinical orthopaedics and related research 2010;468:1498-505.

106.   Meyer DC, Hoppeler H, von Rechenberg B, Gerber C. A pathomechanical concept explains muscle loss and fatty muscular changes following surgical tendon release. Journal of Orthopaedic Research 2004;22:1004-7.

107.   Elliott JM, O'Leary S, Sterling M, Hendrikz J, Pedler A, Jull G. Magnetic resonance imaging findings of fatty infiltrate in the cervical flexors in chronic whiplash. Spine 2010;35(9):948-54.

108.   Elliott JM, Jull G, Noteboom JT, Darnell R, Galloway G, Gibbon WW. Fatty infiltration in the cervical extensor muscles in persistent whiplash-associated disorders: a magnetic resonance imaging analysis. Spine 2006;31:E847-55.

109.   Elliott J, Sterling M, Noteboom JT, Darnell R, Galloway G, Jull G. Fatty infiltrate in the cervical extensor muscles is not a feature of chronic, insidious-onset neck pain. Clinical Radiology 2008;63(6):681-7.

110.   Elliott J, Sterling M, Noteboom JT, Treleaven J, Galloway G, Jull G. The clinical presentation of chronic whiplash and the relationship to findings of MRI fatty infiltrates in the cervical extensor musculature: a preliminary investigation. European Spine Journal 2009;18:1371-8.

111.   Elliott JM. Are there implications for morphological changes in neck muscles after whiplash injury? Spine 2011;36(25 Suppl):S205-S10.

112.   Elliott JM, Jull G, Noteboom JT, Galloway G. MRI study of the cross-sectional area for the cervical extensor musculature in patients with persistent whiplash associated disorders (WAD). Manual Therapy 2008;13:258-65.

113.   Rezasoltani A, Ali-Reza A, Khosro K-K, Abbass R. Preliminary study of neck muscle size and strength measurements in females with chronic non-specific neck pain and healthy control subjects. Manual Therapy 2010;15:400-3.

114.   Armijo-Olivo S, Warren S, Fuentes J, Magee DJ. Clinical relevance vs. statistical significance: Using neck outcomes in patients with temporomandibular disorders as an example. Manual Therapy 2011;16:563-72.

115.   Kristjansson E. Reliability of ultrasonography for the cervical multifidus muscle in asymp-tomatic and symptomatic subjects. Manual Therapy 2004;9:83-8.

116.   Fernández-de-las-Peñas C, Albert-Sanchís JC, Buil M, Benitez JC, Alburquerque-Sendín F. Cross-sectional area of cervical multifidus muscle in females with chronic bilateral neck pain compared to controls. Journal of Orthopaedic & Sports Physical Therapy 2008;38(4):175-80.

117.   De Loose V, Van den Oord M, Keser I, Burnotte F, Van Tiggelen D, Dumarey A et al. MRI study of the morphometry of the cervical musculature in F-16 pilots. Aviation, space, and environmental medicine 2009;80(8):727-31.

118.   Oksanen A, Erkintalo M, Metsähonkala L, Anttila P, Laimi K, Hiekkanen H et al. Neck muscles cross-sectional area in adolescents with and without headache - MRI study. European Journal of Pain 2008;12:952-9.

119.   Elliott JM, Jull G, Noteboom JT, Durbridge GL, Gibbon WW. Magnetic resonance imaging study of cross-sectional area of the cervical extensor musculature in an asymptomatic cohort. Clinical Anatomy 2007;20:35-40.

120.   Uhlig Y, Weber BR, Grob D, Muntener M. Fiber composition and fibre transformations in neck muscles of patients with dysfunction of the cervical spine. Journal of orthopedic research 1995;13:240-9.

121.   Falla D, Rainoldi A, Jull G, Stavrou G, Tsao H. Lack of correlation between sternocleidomastoid and scalene muscle fatigability and duration of symptoms in chronic neck pain patients. Neurophysiologie clinique 2004;34:159-65.

122.   Cagnie B, Barbe T, Vandemæle P, Achten E, Cambier D, Danneels L. MRI analysis of muscle/fat index of the superficial and deep neck muscles in an asymptomatic cohort. European Spine Journal 2009;18:704-9.

123. Woodhouse A, Vasseljen O. Altered motor control patterns in whiplash and chronic neck pain. BMC Musculoskeletal Disorders 2008;9:90.

124. Cagnie B, O'Leary S, Elliott J, Peeters I, Parlevliet T, Danneels L. Pain-induced changes in the activity of the cervical extensor muscles evaluated by muscle functional magnetic resonance imaging. Clinical Journal of Pain 2011;27:392-7.

125. Stokes M, Hides J, Elliott JM, Kiesel K, Hodges PW. Rehabilitative ultrasound imaging of the posterior paraspinal muscles. Journal of Orthopaedic & Sports Physical therapy, 2007;37(10):581-95.

126. Sommerich CM, Joines SMB, Hermans V, Moon SD. Use of surface electromyography to estimate neck muscle activity. Journal of Elektromyography and Kinesiology 2000;10:377-98.

127. Vasavada AN, Siping L, Scott D. Influence of muscle morphometry and moment arms on the moment-generating capacity of human neck muscles. Spine 1998;23(4):412-22.

128. Drake RL, Vogl WA, Mitchell AWM. Gray's Anatomy for students. 2 ed. Philadelphia: Churchill Livingstone Elsevier; 2010.

129. Tillmann BN. Atlas der Anatomie des Menschen. Berlin, Heidelberg, New York: Springer Verlag; 2005.

130. Leonhard H, Tillmann B, Töndury G, Zilles K, editors. Rauber / Kopsch, Anatomie des Menschen, Lehrbuch und Atlas, Band I, Bewegungsapparat. 3 ed. Stuttgart - New York: Georg Thieme Verlag; 2003.

131. Anderson JS, Hsu AW, Vasavada AN. Morphology, architecture, and biomechanics of human cervical multifidus. Spine 2005;30(4):E86-91.

132. Schuenke M, Schulte E, Schumacher U. Thieme Atlas of Anatomy, General Anatomy and Musculoskeletal System. Stuttgart - New York: Georg Thieme Verlag; 2006.

133. Schünke M. Funktionelle Anatomie - Topographie und Funktion des Bewegungssystems. Stuttgart: Georg Thieme Verlag; 2000.

134. Bergmark A. Stability of the lumbar spine. A study in mechanical engineering. Acta orthopaedica Scandinavica Suppl 1989;230:1-54.

135. Boyd-Clark LC, Briggs CA, Galea MP. Comparative histochemical composition of muscle fibres in a pre- and postvertebral muscle of the cervical spine. Journal of Anatomy 2001;199:709-16.

136. Cholewicki J, McGill SM. Mechanical stability of the in vivo lumbar spine: inplications for injury and chronic low back pain. Clinical Biomechanics 1996;11(1):1-15.

137. Conley MS, Stone MH, Nimmons M, Dudley GA. Resistance training and human cervical muscle recruitment plasticity. Journal of Applied Physiology 1997;83:2105-11.

138. Peolsson A, Brodin L-Å, Peolsson M. A tissue velocity ultrasound imaging investigation of the dorsal neck muscles during resisted isometric extension. Manual Therapy 2010.

139. Cagnie B, Dolphens M, Peeters I, Achten E, Cambier D, Danneels L. Use of muscle functional magnetic resonance imaging to compare cervical flexor

activity between patients with whiplash-associated disorders and people who are healthy. Physical Therapy 2010;90(8):1157-64.

140.   English AWM, Wolf SL. The motor unit. Physical Therapy 1982;62(12):1763-72.

141.   De Luca CJ, Forrest WJ. Some properties of motor unit action potential trains recorded during constant force isometric contractions in man. Kybernetik 1973;12:160-8.

142.   Semmler JG, Nordstrom MA, Wallace CJ. Relationship between motor unit short-term synchronization and common drive in human first dorsal interosseous muscle. Brain Research 1997;767:314-20.

143.   Lemon RN. Decending pathways in motor control. Annual review of neuroscience 2008;31:195-218.

144.   Lemon RN, Griffith J. Comparing the function of the corticospinal system in different species: organizational differences for motor specialization? . Muscle Nerve 2005;32:261-79.

145.   Farmer SF, Swash M, Ingram DA, Stephens JA. Changes in motor unit synchronization following central nervous lesions in man. Journal of Physiology 1993;463:83-105.

146.   Negro F, Farina D. Linear transmission of cortical oscillations to the neural drive to muscles is mediated by common projections to populations of motor neurons in humans. The Journal of Physiology 2011;589(3):629-37.

147.   Enoka RM, Baudry S, Rudroff T, Farina D, Klass M. Unraveling the neurophysiology of muscle fatigue. Journal of Electromyography and Kinesiology 2011;21:208-19.

148.   Treleaven J. Sensorimotor disturbances in neck disorders affecting postural stability, head and eye movement control. Manual Therapy 2008;13:2-11.

149.   Caneiro JP, O'Sullivan P, Burnett A, Barach A, OÄNeil D, Tveit O. The influence of different sitting postures on head/neck posture and muscle activity. Manual Therapy 2010;15(1):54-60.

150.   Falla D, O'Leary S, Fagan AE, Jull G. Recruitment of the deep cervical flexor muscles during a postural-correction exercise performed in sitting. Manual Therapy 2007;12:139-43.

151.   English AWM, Wolf SL, Segal RL. Compartmentalization of muscles and their motor nuclei: the partitioning hypothesis. Physical Therapy 1993;73:857-67.

152.   Sanders DB, Stalberg EV, Nandedkar SD. Analysis of the electromyographic interference pattern. Journal of Clinical Neurophysiology 1996;13(5):385-400.

153.   Stashuk D. EMG signal decomposition: how can it be accomplished and used? Journal of Electromyography and Kinesiology 2001;11:151-73.

154.   Merletti R, Farina D. Analysis of intramuscular electromyogram signals. Philosophical transactions of the royal society A 2009;367:357-68.

155.   Daube JR, Rubin DI. Needle electromyography. Muscle Nerve 2009;39:244-70.

156.   Dideriksen JL, Farina D, Baekgaard M, Enoka RM. An integrative model of motor unit activity during sustained submaximal contractions. Journal of Applied Physiology 2010;108:1550-62.

157.   Farina D, Merletti R, Enoka RM. The extraction of neural strategies from the surface EMG. Journal of Applied Physiology 2004;96:1486-95.
158.   Dimitrova NA, Dimitrov GV. Interpretation of EMG changes with fatigue: facts, pitfalls, and fallacies. Journal of Electromyography and Kinesiology 2003;13:13-36.
159.   Dideriksen JL, Falla D, Bækgaard M, Mogensen ML, Steimle KL, Farina D. Comparison between the degree of motor unit short-term synchronization and recurrence quantification analysis of the surface EMG in two human muscles. Clinical Neurophysiology 2009;120(12):1086-2092.
160.   Holobar A, Farina D, Gazzoni M, Merletti R, Zazula D. Estimating motor unit discharge patterns from high-density surface electromyogram. Clinical Neurophysiology 2009;120:551-62.
161.   McGill KC, Lateva ZC, Marateb HR. EMGLAB: an interactive EMG decomposition program. Journal of Neuroscience Methods 2005;149:121-33.
162.   Sale DG. Influence of exercise and training on motor unit activation Exercise and sport sciences reviews 1987;15:95-151.
163.   Matthews PBC. Relationship of firing intervals of human motor units to the trajectory of post-spike after-hyperpolarization and synaptic noise. Journal of Physiology 1996;492(2):597-628.
164.   Semmler JG, Nordstrom MA. Motor unit discharge and force tremor in skilland strength-trained individuals. Experimental Brain Research 1998;119:27-38.
165.   Moritz CT, Barry BK, Pascoe MA, Enoka RM. Discharge rate variability influences the variation in force fluctuations across the working range of a hand muscle. Journal of Neurophysiology 2004;93:2449-59.
166.   Henneman E. The size-principle: a deterministic output emerges from a set of probabilistic connections. The Journal of experimental biology 1985;115:105-12.
167.   Henneman E. Relation between size of neurons and their susceptibility to discharge. Science 1957;126(3287):1345-7.
168.   Garnett R, Stephens JA. Changes in the recruitment threshold of motor units produced by cutaneous stimulation in man. Journal of Physiology 1981;311:463-73.
169.   De Luca CJ, Roy AM, Erim Z. Synchronization of motor-unit fireings in several human muscles. Journal of Neurophysiology 1993;70(5):2010-23.
170.   Moore GP, Segundo JP, Perkel DH, Levitan H. Statistical signs of synaptic interaction in neurons. Biophysical Journal 1970;10:876-900.
171.   Semmler JG. Motor unit synchronization and neuromuscular performance. Exercise and sport sciences reviews 2002;30(1):8-14.
172.   Nordstrom MA, Fuglevand AJ, Enoka RM. Estimating the strength of common input to human motoneurons from the cross-correlogram. Journal of Physiology 1992;453:547-74.
173.   Farina D, Negro F, Gizzi L, Falla D. Low-frequency oscillations of the neural drive to the muscle are increased with experimental muscle pain. Journal of Neurophysiology 2012;107(3):958-65.

174. Ellaway PH. Cumulative sum technique and its application to the analysis of peristimulus time histograms. Electroencephalography and clinical neurophysiology 1978;45(2):302-4.

175. Davey NJ, Ellaway PH, Stein RB. Statistical limits for detecting change in the cumulative sum derivative of the peristimulus time histogram. Journal of Neuroscience Methods 1986;17:153-66.

176. Rosenberg JR, Amjad AM, Breeze P, Brillinger DR, Halliday DM. The Fourier approach to the identification of functional coupling between neuronal spike trains. Progress in biophysics and molecular biology 1989;53:1-31.

177. Negro F. Population coding of neural drive in human motor units during voluntary isometric contractions. Aalborg, Denmark: Aalborg University; 2010.

178. Rosenberg JR, Amjad AM, P B, Brillinger DR, Halliday DM. The fourier approach to the identification of functional coupling between neuronal spike trains. Progress in biophysics and molecular biology 1989;53:1-31.

179. Passatore M, Roatta S. Înfluence of sympathetic nervous system on sensorimotor function: whiplash associated disorders (WAD) as a model. European Journal of Applied Physiology 2006;98:423-49.

180. Sjölander P, Michaelson P, Jaric S, Djupsjöbacka M. Sensorimotor disturbances in chronic neck pain--range of motion, peak velocity, smoothness of movement, and repositioning acuity. Manual Therapy 2008;13(2):122-31.

181. Siegmund GP, Blouin J-S, Brault JR, Hedenstierna S, Inglis JT. Electromyography of superficial and deep neck muscles during isometric, voluntary, and reflex contractions. Journal of Biomechanical Engineering 2007;129(1):66-77.

182. Lee JP, Tseng WY, Shau YW, Wang CL, Wang HK, F WS. Measurement of segmental cervical multifidus contraction by ultrasonography in asymptomatic adults. Manual Therapy 2007;12:286-94.

183. Javanshir K, Amiri M, Mohnseni-Bandpei MA, Rezasoltani A, Fernández-de-las-Peñas C. Ultrasonography of the cervical muscles: a critical review of the literature. Journal of Manipulative and Physiological Therapeutics 2010;33:630-7.

184. Whittaker JL, Teyhen DS, Elliott JM, Cook K, Langevin HM, Dahl HH et al. Rehabilitative ultrasound imaging: understanding the technology and its applications. Journal of Orthopaedic & Sports Physical Therapy 2007;37(8):434-49.

185. Cagnie B, Derese E, Vandamme L, Verstraete K, Cambier D, Danneels L. Validity and reliability of ultrasonography for the longus colli in asymptomatic subjects. Manual Therapy 2009;14:421-6.

186. Dupont A-C, Sauerbrei EE, Fenton PV, Shragge PC, E LG, Richmond FJR. Real-time sonography to estimate muscle thickness: comparison with MRI and CT. Journal of Clinical Ultrasound 2001;29:230-6.

187. Kramer M, Schmid I, Sander S, Högel J, Eisele R, Kinzl L et al. Guidelines for the intramuscular positioning of EMG electrodes in the semispinalis capitis and cervicis muscles. Journal of Electromyography and Kinesiology 2003;13:289-95.

188.   Kramer M. Kinesiologisches fine-wire EMG des m. semispinalis capitis zur   Darstellung   muskulärer   Dysfunktionen   nach   HWS-Beschleunigungsverletzungen II°. Ulm (Germany): Universität Ulm; 2004.
189.   Thiel W. Photographischer Atlas der praktischen Anatomie. 2. ed. Heidelberg: Springer Verlag; 2003.
190.   Schünke M, Schulte E, Schumacher U. Prometheus, LernAtlas der Anatomie. Stuttgart, New York: Georg Thieme Verlag; 2005.
191.   Fernández-de-las-Peñas C, Bueno A, Ferrando J, Elliott JM, Cuadrado MI, Pareja JA. Magnetic resonance imaging study of the morphometry of cervical extensor muscles in chronic tension-type headache. Chephalalgia 2007;27:355-62.
192.   Hides J, Gilmore C, Stanton W, Bohlscheid E. Multifidus size and symmetry among chronic LBP and healthy asymptomatic subjects. Manual Therapy 2008;13:43-9.
193.   Wallwork TL, Stanton WR, Freke M, Hides JA. The effect of chronic low back pain on size and contraction of the lumbar multifidus muscle. Manual Therapy 2009;14(5):496-500.
194.   Jull G, Bogduk N, Marsland A. A. The accuracy of manual diagnosis for cervical zygapophysial joint pain syndromes. The Medical journal of Australia 1988;148(5):233-6.
195.   Jensen K, Andersen HØ, Olesen J, Lindblom U. Pressure-pain threshold in human temporal region. Evaluation of a new pressure algometer. Pain 1986;25:313-23.
196.   Nussbaum EL, Daownes L. Reliability of clinical pressure-pain algometric measurments obtained on consecutive days. Physical Therapy 1998;78(2):160-9.
197.   Kinser AM, Sands WA, Stone MH. Reliability and validity of a pressure algometer. Journal of Strength and Conditioning Research 2009;23(1):312-4.
198.   Keating L, Lubke C, Powell V, Young T, Souvlis T, Jull G. Mid-thoracic tenderness: a comparison of pressure pain threshold between spinal regions, in asymptomatic subjects. Manual Therapy 2001;6(1):34-9.
199.   Schenk P, Laeubli t, Klipstein A. Validity of pressure pain thresholds in female workers with and without recurrent low back pain. European Spine Journal 2007;16:267-75.
200.   Shiau YY, Peng CC, Wen SC, Lin LD, Wang JS, Lou KL. The effects of masseter muscle pain on biting performance. Journal of Oral Rehabilitation 2003;30:978-84.
201.   Walton D, MacDermid J, Nielson W, Teasell R, Reese H, Levesque L. Pressure pain threshold testing demonstrateds predictive ability in people with cute whiplash. Journal of Orthopaedic & Sports Physical Therapy 2011;41(9):658-65.
202.   Walton D, MacDermid J, Nielson W, Teasell R, Nailer T, Maheu P. A descriptive study of pressure pain threshold at 2 standardized sites in people with acute or subacute neck pain. Journal of Orthopaedic & Sports Physical Therapy 2011;41(9):651-7.
203.   Williamson A, Hoggart B. Pain: a review of three commonly used pain rating scales. Journal of Clinical Nursing 2005;14:798-804.

204.   Jensen MP, Turner JA, Romano JM, D FL. Comparative reliability and validity of chronic pain intensity measures. Pain 1999;83:157-62.
205.   Williams ACdC, Davies HTO, Chadury Y. Simple pain rating scales hide complex idiosyncratic meanings. Pain 2000;85:457-63.
206.   Gridley L, van den Dolder PA. The percentage improvement in pain scale as a measure of physiotherapy treatment effects. Australian Journal of Physiotherapy 2001;47:133-6.
207.   Rosier EM, Iadarola MJ, Coghill RC. Reproducibility of pain measurement and pain perception. Pain 2002;98:205-16.
208.   Jensen MP, McFarland CA. Increasing the reliability and validity of pain intensity measurement in chronic pain patients. Pain 1993;55:195-203.
209.   Price DD, Bush FM, Long S, Harkins SW. A comparison of pain measurement characteristics of mechanical visual analogue and simple numerical rating scales. Pain 1994;56:217-26.
210.   Myles PS, Troedel S, Boquest M, Reeves M. The pain visual analog scale: Is it linear or nonlinear? Anesthesia and Analgesia 1999;89:1517-20.
211.   Dexter F, Chestnug DH. Analysis of statistcal tests to compare visual analog scale measurements among groups [clinical investiation]. Anesthesiology 1995;82(4):896-902.
212.   Abrams D, Davidson M, Harrick J, Harcourt P, Hylinski, Maria, Clancy J. Monitoring the change: Current trends in outcome measure usage in physiotherapy. Manual Therapy 2006;11:46-53.
213.   Schomacher J. Gütekriterien der visuellen Analogskala zur Schmerzbewertung. Physioscience 2008;4:125-33.
214.   MacDermid JC, Walton DM, Avery S, Blanchard A, Etruw E, McAlpine C et al. Measurement properties of the neck disability index: a systematic review. Journal of Orthopaedic & Sports Physical Therapy 2009;39(5):400-17.
215.   Young BA, Walkter MJ, Strunce JB, Boyles RE, Whitman JM, Childs JD. Responsiveness of the neck disability index in patients with mechanical neck disorders. The Spine Journal 2009;9:802-8.
216.   Vernon H. The neck disability index: state-of-the-art, 1991-2008. Journal of Manipulative and Physiological Therapeutics 2008;31:491-502.
217.   Vernon H, Mior S. The neck disability index: a study of reliability and validity. Journal of Manipulative and Physiological Therapeutics 1991;14(7):409-15.
218.   McCarthy MJH, Grevitt MP, Silcocks P, Hobbs G. The reliability of the Vernon and Mior neck disability index, and its validity compared with the short form-36 health survey questionnaire. European Spine Journal 2007;16:2111-7.
219.   Hermann KM, Reese CS. Relationsship among selected measures of impairment, functional limitation, and disability in patients with cervical spine disorders. Physical Therapy 2001;81(3):903-14.
220.   Riddle DL, Stratford PW. Specific functional status measures of patients with cervical spine disorders. Physical Therapy 1998;78(9):951-63.
221.   Cleland JA, Fritz JM, Whitman JM, Palmer JA. The reliability and construct validity of the neck disability index and patient specific functional scale in patients with cervical radiculopathy. Spine 2006;31(5):598-602.

222. Kasi PK. Characterization of motor unit discharge rate in patients with amytrophic lateral sclerosis (ALS). Worcester (USA): Worcester Polytechnic Institute; 2009.

223. Kukulka CG, Clamann HP. Comparison of the recruitment and discharge properties of motor units in human brachial biceps and adductor pollicis during isometric contractions. Brain Research 1981;219:45-55.

224. Christou EA, Rudroff T, Enoka JA, Meyer F, Enoka RM. Discharge rate during low-force isometric contractions infuences motor unit coherence below 15 Hz but not motor unit synchronization. Experimental Brain Research 2007;178:285-95.

225. Holobar A, Minetto MA, Botter A, Negro F, Farina D. Experimental analysis of accuracy in the identification of motor unit spike trains from hig-density surface EMG. IDEE Transactions on Neural Systems and Rehabilitation Engineering 2010;18(3):221-9.

226. Falla D, Farina D. Motor units in cranial and caudal regions of the upper trapezius muscle have different discharge rates during brief static contractions. Acta Physiologica 2008;192:551-8.

227. Falla D, Farina D. Non-uniform adaptation of motor unit discharge rates during sustained static contraction of the upper trapezius muscle. Experimental Brain Research 2008;191:363-70.

228. Keen DA, Fuglevand AJ. Common input to motor neurons innervating the same and different compartments of the human extensor digitorum muscle. Journal of Neurophysiology 2004;91:55-62.

229. Reilly KT, Nordstrom MA, Schieber MH. Short-term synchronization between motor units in different functional subdivisions of the human flexor digitorum profundus muscle. Journal of Neurophysiology 2004;92:734-42.

230. McIsaac TL, Fuglevand AJ. Motor-unit synchrony within and across compartments of the human flexor digitorum superficialis. Journal of Neurophysiology 2006;97:550-6.

231. Hudson AL, Gandevia SC, Butler JE. Common rostrocaudal gradient of output from human intercostal motoneurones during voluntary and automatic breathing. Respiratory physiology & neurobiology 2011;175(1):20-8.

232. De Troyer A, Gorman RB, Gandevia SC. Distribution of inspiratory drive to the external intercostal muscles in humans. Journal of Physiology 2003;546(3):943-54.

233. Lee PJ, Rogers EL, Granata KP. Active trunk stiffness increases with co-contraction. Journal of Elektromyography and Kinesiology 2006;16:51-7.

234. Fernández-de-las-Peñas C, Falla D, Arendt-Nielsen L, Farina D. Cervical muscle co-activation in isometric contractions is enhanced in chronic tension-type headache patients. Chephalalgia 2008;28:744-51.

235. Javanshir K, Ortega-Santiago R, Mohseni-Bandpei MA, Miangolarra-Page JC, Fernández-de-las-Peñas C. Exploration of somatosensory impairments in subjects with mechanical idiopathick neck pain: a preliminary study. Journal of Manipulative and Physiological Therapeutics 2010;33:493-9.

236.   Kasch H, Stengaard-Pedersen K, Arendt-Nielsen L, Staehelin Jensen T. Pain thresholds and tenderness in neck and head following acute whiplash injury: a prospective study. Cephalgia 2001;21(3):189-97.
237.   Kamper SJ, Maher CG, Hush JM, Pedler A, Sterling M. Relationship between pressure pain thresholds and pain ratings in patients with whiplash-associated disorders. Clinical Journal of Pain 2011;27:495-501.
238.   Wolf HD. Bewegungssegment C2/3 - auch eine Übergangsregion der Wirbelsäule. Manuelle Medizin 1997;35:59-62.
239.   Lund JP, Donga R, Widmer CG, Stohler CS. The pain-adaptation model: a discussion of the relationship between musculoskeletal pain and motor activity. Canadian Journal of Physiology and Pharmacology 1991;49:683-94.
240.   Arendt-Nielsen L, Graven-Nielsen T. Muscle pain: Sensory implications and interaction with motor control. Clinical Journal of Pain 2008;24:291-8.
241.   Birch L, Christensen H, Arendt-Nielsen L, Graven-Nielsen T, Søgaard K. The influence of experimental muscle pain on motor unit activity during low-level contraction. European Journal of Applied Physiology 2000;83:200-6.
242.   Falla D, Farina D. Neural and muscular factors associated with motor impairment in neck pain. Current Rheumatology Reports 2007;9:497-502.
243.   Graven-Nielsen T, Svensson P, Arendt-Nielsen L. Effects of experimental muscle pain on muscle activity and co-ordination during static and dynamic motor function. Electroencephalography and clinical Neurophysiology 1997;10:156-64.
244.   Grimsby O, Rivard J. Exercise Biomechanics. In: Grimsby O, Rivard J, editors. Science, theory and clinical application in orthopaedic manual physical therapy, Applied science and theory. Taylorsville, UT: The Academy of Graduate Physical Therapy, Inc.; 2008. p 243-84.
245.   Elliott JM, O'Leary SP, Cagnie B, Durbridge G, Danneels L, Jull G. Craniocervical orientation affects muscle activation when exercising the cervical extensors in healthy subjects. Archives of Physical Medicine and Rehabilitation 2010;91:1418-22.
246.   Panjabi MM. The stabilizing system of the spine. Part I. Function, dysfunction, adaptation, and enhancement. Journal of spinal disorders & techniques 1992;5(4):383-9.
247.   White AA, Panjabi MM. Clinical biomechanics of the spine. Philadelphia ... J. B. Lippincott Company; 1990.
248.   ter Haar Romeny BM, Denier van der Gon JJ, Gelen CC. Changes in recruitment order of motor units in the human biceps muscle. Experimental Neurology 1982;78(2):360-8.
249.   ter Haar Romeny BM, van der Gon JJ, Gielen CC. Relation between location of a motor unit in the human biceps brachii and its critical firing levels for different tasks. Experimental Neurology 1984;85(3):631-50.
250.   De Troyer A, Kirkwood PA, Wilson TA. Respiratory action of the intercostal muscles. Physiological Reviews 2005;85:717-56.
251.   Butler JE, Gandevia SC. The output from human inspiratory motoneurone poos. Journal of Physiology 2008;586(5):1257-64.
252.   Butler JE. Drive to the human respiratory muscles. Respiratory physiology & neurobiology 2007;159(2):115-26.

253. Arendt-Nielsen L, Falla D. Motor control adjustments in musculoskeletal pain and the implications for pain recurrence. Pain 2009;142:171-2.

254. Szeto GPY, Straker LM, O'Sullivan PB. A comparison of symptomatic and asymptomatic office workers performing monotonous keyboard work – 2: Neck and shoulder kinematics. Manual Therapy 2005;10:281-91.

255. Johansson H, Sojka P. Pathophysiological mechanisms involved in genesis and spread of muscular tension in occupational muscle pain and in chronic musculoskeletal pain syndromes: a hypothesis. Medical Hypotheses 1991;35:196-203.

256. Lee H, Nicholson LL, Adams RD. Cervical range of motion associations with subclinical pain. Spine 2003;29(1):33-40.

257. Röijezon U, Björklund M, Djupsjöbacka M. The slow and fast components of postural sway in chronic neck pain. Manual Therapy 2011;16:273-8.

258. Treleaven J, Jull G, Grip H. Head eye co-ordination and gaze stability in subjects with persistent whiplash associated disorders. Manual Therapy 2011;16:252-7.

259. Roatta S, Arendt-Nielsen L, Farina D. Sympathetic-induced changes in discharge rate and spike-triggered average twitch torque of low-threshold motor units in humans. The Journal of Physiology 2008;586(22):5561-74.

260. Boudreau S, Farina D, Djupsjöbacka M, Falla D. Sympathetic activation impairs proprioceptive acuity of the neck. The XVIII International Conference of the Society of Electrophysiology and Kinesiology (ISEK). Aalborg (Denmark); 2010.

261. Sjøgaard G, Lundberg U, Kadefors R. The role of muscle activity and mental load in the development of pain and degenerative processes ant the muscle cel level during computer work. European Journal of Applied Physiology 2000;83:99-105.

262. Rosendahl L, Larsson B, Kristiansen J, Peolsson M, Søgaard K, Kjaer M et al. Increase in muscle nociceptive substances and anaerobic metabolism in patients with trapezius myalgia: microdialysis in rest and during exercise. Pain 2004;112:324-34.

263. Kristjansson E, Leivseth G, Brinckmann P, Frobin W. Increased sagittal plane segmental motion in the lower cervical spine in women with chronic whiplash-associated disorders, grades I-II. Spine 2003;28(19):2215-21.

264. Cleland JA, Childs JD, Fritz JM, Whitman JM. Interrater reliability of the history and physical examination in patients with mechanical neck pain. Archives of Physical Medicine and Rehabilitation 2006;87:1388-95.

265. Olson KA, Joder D. Diagnosis and treatment of cervical spine clinical instability. Journal of Orthopaedic & Sports Physical Therapy 2001;31(4):194-206.

266. Niere KR, Torney SK. Clinicians' perceptions of minor cervical instability. Manual Therapy 2004;9:144-50.

267. Jull G. Übungsansatz bei HWS-Störungen: Wie fließen die Ergebnisse der Forschung in die Praxis ein? . Manuelle Therapie 2009;13(3):110-6.

268.   O'Leary S, Falla D, Jull G, Vicenzino B. Muscle specificity in tests of cervical flexor muscle performance. Journal of Elektromyography and Kinesiology 2007;17:35-40.

269.   Cibulka MT. Sternocleidomastoid muscle imbalance in a patient with recurrent headache. Manual Therapy 2006;11:78-82.

270.   Sarig-Bahat H. Evidence for exercise therapy in mechanical neck disorders. Manual Therapy 2003;8(1):10-20.

271.   Bronfort G, Evans R, Nelson B, Aker PD, Goldsmith CH, Vernon H. A randomized clinical trial of exercise and spinal manipulation for patients with chronic neck pain. Spine 2001;26:788-97.

272.   Evans R, Bronfort G, Nelson B, Goldsmith CH. Two-year folow-up of a randomized clinical trial of spinal manipulation and two types of exercise for patients with chronic neck pain. Spine 2002;27(21):2383-9.

273.   Falla D, Jull G, Hodges PW, Vicenzino B. An endurance-strength training regime is effective in reduction manifestations of cervical flexor muscle fatigue in females with chronic neck pain. Clinical Neurophysiology 2006;117:828-37.

274.   Ylinen J, Takala E-P, Kautiainen H, Nykänen M, Häkkinen AH, Pohjolainen T et al. Effect of long-term neck muscle training on pressure pain threshold: A randomized controlled trial. European Journal of Pain 2005;9:673-81.

275.   Falla D, Jull G, Hodges PW. Training the cervical muscles with prescribed motor tasks does not change muscle activation during a functional activity. Manual Therapy 2008;13:507-12.

276.   Schomacher J. Physiotherapeutische Tests zur Symptomlokalisation im HWS-Bereich, Teil 1. Manuelle Therapie 2006;10(2):60-8.

277.   Schomacher J. Physiotherapeutische Tests zur Symptomlokalisation im HWS-Bereich, Teil 2. Manuelle Therapie 2006;10(3):108-18.

278.   Conley MS, Stone MH, Nimmons M, Dudley GA. Specificity of resistance training responses in neck muscle size and strength. European Journal of Applied Physiology 1997;76:443-8.

279.   Hollmann W. Training, Grundlagen und Anpassungsprozesse. Studienbrief der Trainerakademie Köln des Deutschen Sportbundes 9. Schondorf: Hofmann-Verlag; 1990.

280.   Aquino RL, Caires PM, Furtado FC, Loureiro AV, Ferreira PH, Ferreira ML. Applying joint mobilization ad different cervical vertebral levels does not influence immediate pain reduction in patients with chronic neck pain: a randomized clinical trial. Journal of Manual & Manipulative Therapy 2009;17(2):95-100.

281.   Schomacher J, Learman K. Symptom Localization Tests in the Cervical Spine: A Descriptive Study using Imaging Verification. Journal of Manual & Manipulative Therapy 2010;18(2):97-101.

282.   Cleland JA, Glynn P, Whitman JM, Eberhart SL, MacDonald C, Childs JD. Short-term effects of thrust versus nonthrust mobilization/manipulation directed at the thoracic spine in patients with neck pain: a randomized clinical trial. Physical Therapy 2007;87(4):431-40.

283.   Haas M, Groupp E, Panzer D, Partna L, Lumsden S, Aickin M. Efficacy of cervical endplay assessment as an indicator for spinal manipulation. Spine 2003;29(11):1091-6.

Paper 1 to 4

The following pages contain the original studies on which this thesis is based. These are reprinted here with permission from the publishers.

Paper 1:
Schomacher J, Dideriksen J L, Farina D, Falla D. Recruitment of motor units in two fascicles of the semispinalis cervicis muscle. The Journal of Neurophysiology, 2012; 107(11): 3078-3085 / doi: 10.1152/jn.00953.2011.

Paper 2:
Schomacher J, Farina D, Lindstroem R, Falla D. Chronic trauma-induced neck pain impairs the neural control of the deep semispinalis cervicis muscle. Clinical Neurophysiology, 123(7), 2012: 1403-1408 / doi: 10.1016/j.clinph.2011.11.033.

Paper 3:
Schomacher J, Boudreau S A, Petzke F, Falla D. Localized pain sensitivity is associated with reduced activation of the semispinalis cervicis muscle in patients with neck pain. Clinical Journal of Pain. 2013 Jan 30. [Epub ahead of print]

Paper 4:
Schomacher J, Petzke F, Falla D. Localised resistance selectively activates the semispinalis cervicis muscle in patients with neck pain. Manual Therapy, 2012 Dec;17(6):544-548 / doi: 10.1016/j.math.2012.05.012.

Recruitment of motor units in two fascicles of the semispinalis cervicis muscle

Jochen Schomacher, Jakob Lund Dideriksen, Dario Farina and Deborah Falla

J Neurophysiol 107:3078-3085, 2012. First published 7 March 2012;
doi: 10.1152/jn.00953.2011

Journal of Neurophysiology publishes original articles on the function of the nervous system. It is published 24
times a year (twice monthly) by the American Physiological Society, 9650 Rockville Pike, Bethesda MD
20814-3991. Copyright © 2012 the American Physiological Society. ESSN: 1522-1598. Visit our website at
http://www.the-aps.org/.

J Neurophysiol 107: 3078–3085, 2012.
First published March 7, 2012; doi:10.1152/jn.00953.2011.

Recruitment of motor units in two fascicles of the semispinalis cervicis muscle

Jochen Schomacher,[1] Jakob Lund Dideriksen,[1] Dario Farina,[2] and Deborah Falla[2,3]

[1]*Center for Sensory-Motor Interaction (SMI), Department of Health Science and Technology, Aalborg University, Aalborg, Denmark; and* [2]*Department of Neurorehabilitation Engineering, Bernstein Focus Neurotechnology Göttingen, Bernstein Center for Computational Neuroscience, University Medical Center Göttingen, Georg-August University, and* [3]*Pain Clinic, Center for Anesthesiology, Emergency and Intensive Care Medicine, University Hospital Göttingen, Göttingen, Germany*

Submitted 24 October 2011; accepted in final form 6 March 2012

Schomacher J, Dideriksen JL, Farina D, Falla D. Recruitment of motor units in two fascicles of the semispinalis cervicis muscle. *J Neurophysiol* 107: 3078–3085, 2012. First published March 7, 2012; doi:10.1152/jn.00953.2011.—This study investigated the behavior of motor units in the semispinalis cervicis muscle. Intramuscular EMG recordings were obtained unilaterally at levels C2 and C5 in 15 healthy volunteers (8 men, 7 women) who performed isometric neck extensions at 5%, 10%, and 20% of the maximal force [maximum voluntary contraction (MVC)] for 2 min each and linearly increasing force contractions from 0 to 30% MVC over 3 s. Individual motor unit action potentials were identified. The discharge rate and interspike interval variability of the motor units in the two locations did not differ. However, the recruitment threshold of motor units detected at C2 ($n = 16$, mean $\pm$ SD: 10.3 $\pm$ 6.0% MVC) was greater than that of motor units detected at C5 ($n = 92$, 6.9 $\pm$ 4.3% MVC) ($P < 0.01$). A significant level of short-term synchronization was identified in 246 of 307 motor unit pairs when computed within one spinal level but only in 28 of 110 pairs of motor units between the two levels. The common input strength, which quantifies motor unit synchronization, was greater for pairs within one level (0.47 $\pm$ 0.32) compared with pairs between levels (0.09 $\pm$ 0.07) ($P < 0.05$). In a second experiment on eight healthy subjects, interference EMG was recorded from the same locations during a linearly increasing force contraction from 0 to 40% MVC and showed significantly greater EMG amplitude at C5 than at C2. In conclusion, synaptic input is distributed partly independently and nonuniformly to different fascicles of the semispinalis cervicis muscle.

motoneurons; synchronization

WHEN THE SYNAPTIC INPUT is equally distributed among motoneurons, small-sized motoneurons are recruited before larger ones (Henneman 1957, 1985). However, motoneurons innervating muscle fibers within the same muscle but with different mechanical action may receive different synaptic input that depends on the biomechanical demands. Those fibers that have a mechanical action with greater advantage for the task may be preferentially activated (English et al. 1993; Hudson et al. 2009), so that the recruitment order is task dependent within a muscle. For example, the recruitment of motor units in different regions of the long head of the biceps brachii varies with the relative amount of elbow flexion and forearm supination torque (ter Haar Romeny et al. 1982, 1984). Moreover, a series of studies on inspiratory muscles showed that the recruitment pattern of motor units across inspiratory motoneuron pools follows the mechanical advantage for respiration (Butler 2007;

Butler and Gandevia 2008). Other muscles with complex mechanical actions, such as the trapezius, also display a location-dependent modulation of motor unit discharge rate, likely reflecting spatial dependence in the control of motor units (Falla and Farina 2008a).

It may be expected that motor units are recruited according to their mechanical advantage for muscles with complex architecture and varying mechanical actions for different fascicles of the muscle. The deep spinal muscles are an example of such complexity. They attach directly to several vertebrae and span numerous articulations to control segmental movement and stability (Bergmark 1989).

In the cervical spine, the fascicles of the semispinalis cervicis muscle originate from the transverse processes of the upper five or six thoracic vertebrae and insert on the cervical spinous processes, from the axis to the seventh cervical vertebrae inclusive. Each fascicle spans four to six segments (Drake et al. 2010; Schuenke et al. 2006). The semispinalis cervicis contributes to extension, ipsilateral lateral flexion, and contralateral rotation of the cervical spine (Drake et al. 2010). These functions are applicable to each segment crossed by the muscle fibers. The mechanical load is higher in the lower cervical spine compared with the middle and upper cervical segments because of the longer moment arm; thus caudal fascicles of the semispinalis cervicis are expected to exert more force than cranial fascicles. Because of this difference in mechanical action, we hypothesized that different fascicles within the semispinalis cervicis receive different synaptic input at a given external extension force according to their mechanical advantage and that motor units innervating fascicles with a higher force demand during isometric neck extension are recruited earlier. To test these hypotheses, this study investigated the behavior of individual motor units in two fascicles of the semispinalis cervicis.

METHODS

Subjects. Fifteen healthy subjects [7 women: age (mean $\pm$ SD): 24.1 $\pm$ 2.9 yr, height: 169.5 $\pm$ 4.2 cm, weight: 69.0 $\pm$ 7.1 kg, body mass index (BMI): 24.0 $\pm$ 3.34 kg/m^2; 8 men: age: 24.2 $\pm$ 1.9 yr, height: 184.8 $\pm$ 7.2 cm, weight: 79.7 $\pm$ 13.0 kg, BMI: 23.2 $\pm$ 2.9 kg/m^2] participated in the first experiment, which aimed to identify the discharge patterns of semispinalis cervicis motor units. In addition, a separate group of eight healthy women (age: 26.0 $\pm$ 2.7 yr, height: 167.3 $\pm$ 8.3 cm, weight: 58.3 $\pm$ 7.3 kg, BMI: 20.8 $\pm$ 2.1 kg/m^2) participated in the second experiment, which aimed to measure the interference EMG of the same muscle at the same two locations (see *Procedures* for a detailed description of the 2 experiments). The data from *experiment 2* were also used in a clinical study that compared activity of the semispinalis cervicis muscle in patients with chronic

Address for reprint requests and other correspondence: D. Falla, Dept. of Neurorehabilitation Engineering, Bernstein Center for Computational Neuroscience, University Medical Center Göttingen, Georg-August Univ., Von-Siebold-Str. 4, 37075 Göttingen, Germany (e-mail: deborah.falla@bccn.uni-goettingen.de).

neck pain and healthy control subjects. Since chronic neck pain is more prevalent in women, the study was designed for female subjects only. For both experiments, subjects were included in the study if their age was between 18 and 45 yr and they were free of neck pain, had not had neck surgery, and had no history of neurological disorders.

Ethical approval for the study was granted by the Ethics Committee of Nordjylland, Denmark (ref. N-20090039). Informed written consent was obtained from all participants, and the procedures were conducted in accordance with the Declaration of Helsinki.

Electromyography. Intramuscular EMG signals were recorded from the semispinalis cervicis muscle on the right side at the level of the second and fifth cervical vertebrae (C2 and C5, respectively) with wire electrodes made of Teflon-coated stainless steel (diameter 0.1 mm; A-M Systems, Carlsborg, WA). In the first experiment the recording end of the wire was cut to expose only the cross section in order to detect action potentials of individual motor units. In the second experiment the recording end of the wire was uninsulated for ~3–4 mm. In this way the recordings provided an indication of the global intensity of activity in each fascicle, as opposed to the selective motor unit recordings in the first experiment that allowed the analysis of only a small portion of each fascicle.

Wires were inserted into the muscle via a 27-gauge hypodermic needle. Needle insertion was guided by ultrasound (Bexander et al. 2005) using a 10-MHz linear transducer (Acuson 128 Computed Sonography) (Lee et al. 2007). Ultrasound is a reliable tool to visualize the deep cervical extensors, as shown by measurements of cross-sectional area (Kristjansson 2004; Stokes et al. 2007). Participants were lying prone on a treatment table with the head resting in a neutral position. The spinous process of C2 was located by palpation as the first bony landmark caudal to the occiput (Lee et al. 2007). The seventh cervical vertebrae (C7) was palpated as the most prominent spinous process (Lee et al. 2007; Stokes et al. 2007). The spinous process of C5 was identified by palpation counting downwards from C2 and confirmed by counting upwards from C7.

Cutaneous landmarks were marked with a pen, and points 15 mm lateral to the midline of the C2 and C5 spinous processes were selected as the insertion points for intramuscular EMG recordings from the semispinalis cervicis (Kramer et al. 2003). For insertion of the wire electrode at the level of C2, the ultrasound transducer was placed transversally in the midline over C2 and moved laterally to image the extensor muscles. Identification of echogenic (bright, reflective) laminae and the spinous process provides the main bony landmarks for identifying the cervical extensors, which are separated by echogenic fascia layers (Stokes et al. 2007; Whittaker et al. 2007).

The needle was inserted after identification of the target muscle and disinfection of the skin. The needle containing the wire was inserted vertically into the muscle belly (Kramer et al. 2003), the location confirmed by ultrasonography, and the needle was removed immediately, leaving the wire in the muscle for the duration of the experiment. The end of the wire was hooked to ensure a stable position of the wire at the insertion point. The same procedure was repeated at C5. These procedures ensured that the location of the wires was within two distinct muscle fascicles (Fig. 1).

Intramuscular EMG signals were amplified (amplifier, EMG-USB2, 256-channel EMG amplifier, OT Bioelettronica, Torino, Italy; 500 Hz-5 kHz), sampled at 10,000 Hz, and converted to digital form by a 12-bit analog-to-digital converter. Common reference electrodes were placed around the right and left wrists.

Procedures. For both the first and second experiments, the participants were seated with their head rigidly fixed in a device for the measurement of multidirectional neck force with their back supported, knees and hips in 90° of flexion, torso firmly strapped to the seat back, and hands resting comfortably in their lap (Falla et al. 2010). The device is equipped with eight adjustable contacts that are fastened around the head to stabilize the head and provide resistance during isometric contractions of the neck. The force device is equipped with force transducers (strain gauges) to measure force in the sagittal and

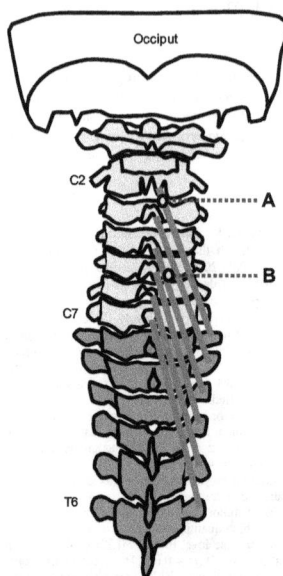

Fig. 1. Schematic representation of the fascicles of the semispinalis cervicis muscle and the insertion points at spinal levels C2 (*A*) and C5 (*B*).

coronal planes. The electrical signals from the strain gauges were amplified (OT Bioelettronica), and their output was displayed on an oscilloscope as visual feedback to the subject.

After a period of familiarization with the measuring device, the subjects performed three neck extension maximum voluntary contractions (MVCs) of 5 s each, separated by 1 min of rest. Verbal encouragement was provided to the subject to promote higher forces in each trial. The highest value of force recorded over the three maximum contractions was selected as the reference MVC. After the MVC contractions the electrodes were inserted as described above. The subject was then seated again in the measuring device with the head and body fixed as described above. In the first experiment the subjects were asked to perform sustained submaximal isometric neck extension contractions for 120 s at 5%, 10%, and 20% MVC. These submaximal force levels were determined in pilot trials as those that allowed identification of single motor unit action potentials with confidence. Each contraction was separated by rest periods of 2 min. After the sustained contractions, three ramp contractions were performed from 0% to 30% MVC over 3 s, with 1 min of rest between contractions.

For the second experiment, the MVCs were performed after wire insertion in order to be able to normalize the EMG amplitude in three subsequent ramped neck extension contractions from 0 to 50% MVC performed over 5 s. For all contractions, the subjects were provided with real-time visual feedback of force on an oscilloscope.

Signal analysis. Single motor unit action potentials were identified from the intramuscular EMG signals of the first experiment with a decomposition algorithm described previously (McGill et al. 2005)

(Fig. 2). The average discharge rate and discharge rate variability (coefficient of variation for interspike interval) were obtained. Motor units that were active for less than half of the duration of the contraction and motor units with repeated inactive periods of several seconds were discarded from the analysis.

From the ramp contractions of the first experiment, the recruitment threshold (expressed as % MVC) of each motor unit was estimated as the force level at which the motor unit began to discharge steadily (i.e., with separation between discharges in the range 20–200 ms). The estimated recruitment threshold values were averaged over the three ramp contractions to reduce variability in estimates. The same motor units were identified across the different recordings by comparing the shapes of the action potentials, obtained from spike-triggered averaging of the high-pass filtered (500 Hz) EMG recording. Action potentials were considered to be generated by the same motor unit if the mean square error between their shapes was <10%.

The level of common input to the motor unit population was assessed in both the time (short-term synchronization) and frequency (coherence) domains for pairs of motor units recorded in the first experiment. Synchronization was evaluated for pairs of units within the individual recording site and for pairs across recording sites. The quality of estimate of the strength of motor unit synchronization from motor units recorded in one single site strongly depends on the accuracy of the decomposition program. The applied decomposition software has been shown to be highly accurate, so that estimates of synchronization from a single electrode site are appropriate (Diderik-sen et al. 2009), as recently discussed (Farina et al. 2012). The degree of motor unit synchronization was estimated by generating cross-histograms (±50 ms relative to the reference motor unit discharge; bin width 1 ms) of all combinations of motor unit pairs (Nordstrom et al. 1992; Semmler et al. 1997). Cross-histograms with an average bin count of <4 were excluded from the analysis (Semmler et al. 1997). The width of the synchronous peak in the cross-histogram was identified with the cumulative sum (Ellaway 1978). Synchronization was quantified by the common input strength (CIS) index (Nordstrom et al. 1992), which denotes the number of synchronous discharges in

excess of chance per second. A significant synchronous peak in the cumulative sum function was defined as an increase of at least 3 standard deviations above the mean of the first 30 bins (Davey et al. 1986). The level of common input was also investigated by coherence analysis between spike trains. The coherence was estimated as the ratio of the squared magnitude of the cross-spectra of two spike trains and the product of their autospectra (Rosenberg et al. 1989). The peak value of coherence in the band 16–32 Hz was used to quantify the strength of common input in the beta band.

Since selective intramuscular EMG signals provide information on a very small muscle portion, we also measured global muscle activity in *experiment 2*. The interference EMG recordings from the second experiment were analyzed by estimating the average rectified value (ARV) from the EMG signals over 300-ms windows in which the average force was 5–40% MVC (5% MVC increments). The ARV computed at these force levels was normalized with respect to the ARV obtained during the MVC. These recordings served to compare the global intensity of muscle activity as a function of force at the two sites (C2 and C5).

Statistical analysis. For the sustained contractions, two-way analysis of variance (ANOVA) was used to test for differences in motor unit discharge rate, coefficient of variation for interspike variability, and synchronization, with spinal level (C2 and C5) and force level (5%, 10%, and 20% MVC) as factors. A one-way ANOVA was used to evaluate differences in motor unit recruitment threshold, CIS, and coherence values within a spinal level compared with motor unit pairs between spinal levels. For comparisons between coherence values, the values were transformed (Amjad et al. 1989) as follows:

$$Z = \arctan h\left(\sqrt{|R_{xy}(\lambda)|^2}\right) \times \sqrt{2N}$$

where $R_{xy}(\lambda)^2$ is the coherence value and N is the number of nonoverlapping signal intervals used for the calculation. Furthermore, a two-way ANOVA was used to examine differences in EMG ARV during the ramped contraction (*experiment 2*) with spinal level (C2 and C5) and force (5–40% MVC in 5% MVC increments) as factors.

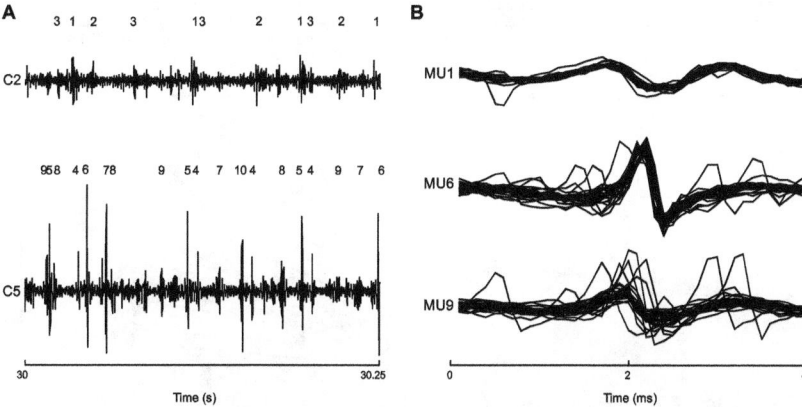

Fig. 2. Result of decomposition of EMG signals during a 10% maximal voluntary contraction (MVC) contraction for a representative subject. In this case, 3 motor units were identified from C2 and 7 from C5. The action potentials from each of these motor units are identified from the intramuscular EMG recording (*A*). *B*: superimposed motor unit action potentials for 3 of the detected motor units. In many cases, not all the identified motor units were included in the analysis since not all were consistently active throughout the contraction. In this example, motor unit (MU)5 and MU10 from C5 were excluded from further analysis since they were active for short periods.

Table 1. *Number of motor units identified and mean discharge rate and coefficient of variation for interspike interval at three force levels*

	5% MVC	10% MVC	20% MVC	Total MUs
Number of MUs				
C2	5	9	13	27
C5	46	57	67	170
Mean discharge rate, pps				
C2	11.3 ± 1.16	12.29 ± 1.91	13.25 ± 4.09	12.57 ± 3.10
C5	9.41 ± 2.91	10.74 ± 4.03	13.80 ± 5.02	11.50 ± 4.54
Coefficient of variation of interspike interval variability				
C2	23.82 ± 5.93	22.18 ± 4.61	23.67 ± 4.87	23.16 ± 4.84
C5	21.97 ± 6.23	23.17 ± 5.99	25.42 ± 5.41	23.75 ± 5.97

Discharge rate and coefficient of variation for interspike interval values are means ± SD. MU, motor unit; MVC, maximal voluntary contraction; pps, pulses per second.

Significant differences revealed by ANOVA were followed by post hoc Student-Newman-Keuls (SNK) pairwise comparisons. Results are reported as means and SD in text and SE in Figs. 5 and 6. Statistical significance was set at $P < 0.05$.

RESULTS

Force. Maximum neck extension force was 214.0 ± 45.0 N for women and 259.1 ± 61.9 N for men in the first experiment. In the second experiment the maximum neck extension force was 187.1 ± 46.1 N.

Motor unit behavior. The discharge patterns of 98 individual motor units were identified across the three submaximal sustained contractions at C5 from the 15 subjects, whereas motor unit activity was detected in 5 of the 15 subjects at C2 (18 motor units in total). Many of these motor units could be tracked over more than one of the sustained contractions. Therefore, in comparisons of motor unit characteristics across force levels some motor units may contribute with values for more than one contraction (and thus the total number is greater than the number of individual motor units). In general, the number of motor units identified increased with increasing force (Table 1).

The discharge rate of the identified motor units was greater at 20% MVC compared with both 10% and 5% MVC ($P < 0.05$) (Table 1 and Fig. 3). The observed mean discharge rate did not differ between C2 and C5 at any force level ($P > 0.05$) (Table 1). The coefficient of variation for the interspike interval (Table 1) did not differ between the two spinal levels or across the three force levels ($P > 0.05$).

The motor unit recruitment thresholds identified from the ramp contractions were determined for 108 of the 116 individual motor units identified during the sustained contractions. The recruitment threshold was significantly greater at C2 ($n = 16$, 10.3 ± 6.0% MVC) compared with C5 ($n = 92$, 6.9 ± 4.3% MVC) ($P < 0.01$), indicating that motor units at C2 were recruited at greater forces than at C5. This result was in agreement with the smaller number of motor units identified at C2 with respect to C5 and with the global EMG amplitude (see below).

Figure 4 illustrates the cross-histograms and cumulative sum functions estimated during a sustained contraction at 10% MVC for a representative subject. In this example, the cross-histograms are shown for two motor unit pairs detected at the C2 level (Fig. 4A) and for two motor unit pairs at the C5 level

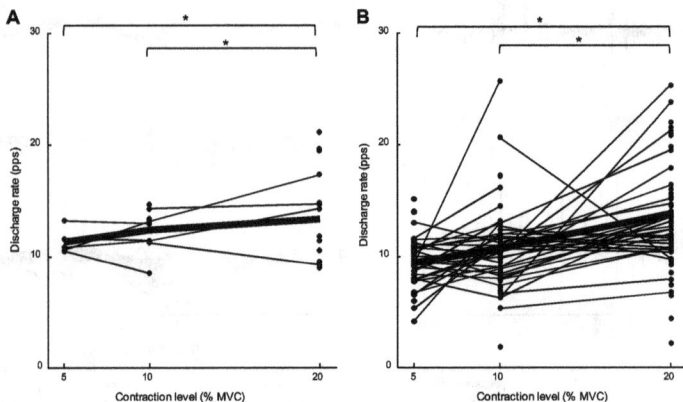

Fig. 3. Average discharge rate for all motor units identified at each contraction force for C2 (*A*) and C5 (*B*), respectively. Lines connect the discharge rates for those motor units that were identified at more than 1 force level. Bold line represents the mean. *$P < 0.05$.

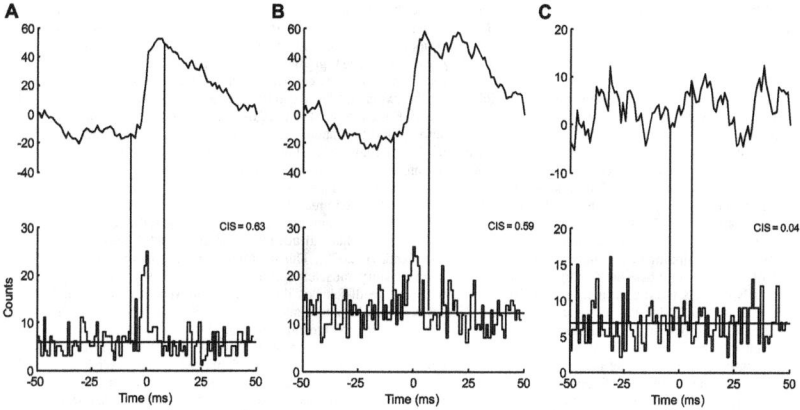

Fig. 4. Representative data showing the cross-histograms and cumulative sum (CuSum) for motor unit pairs in a representative subject during a 10% MVC contraction. The motor unit pairs are detected from the C2 level [A; common input strength (CIS): 0.63], the C5 level (B; CIS: 0.59), and between the 2 levels (C; CIS: 0.04). Vertical lines indicate the boundaries of the synchronous peaks as determined from the CuSum.

(Fig. 4B). Figure 4C shows one motor unit pair across both levels and demonstrates a lower CIS compared with the motor unit pairs within the same spinal level. The peak of the cross-histogram obtained from motor units at different levels was not significant in this example. These observations were confirmed by the group data analysis. The cross-histograms showed significant peaks in 80% of the motor unit pairs (n = 307) when computed within the C2 and C5 levels (89.7% at C2 and 70.4% at C5) but only in 25% of the pairs (n = 110) when computed between levels. Moreover, for these pairs with significant peaks in the cross-histograms, the level of synchronization was significantly greater (P < 0.05) within levels (CIS = 0.48 ± 0.15 for C2; 0.47 ± 0.35 for C5) compared with pairs between levels (0.09 ± 0.07) (Fig. 5). The level of synchronization of these motor unit pairs did not differ between levels (P = 0.91).

For the frequency band 16–32 Hz, the coherence was greater for motor unit pairs from the same level (nontransformed values 0.17 ± 0.13 and 0.19 ± 0.19, respectively) than for motor pairs from different levels (nontransformed value 0.04 ± 0.02) (P < 0.05). Significant coherence was found in 90% of the cases for motor unit pairs from the same level but only in 29% of the cases for motor unit pairs from different levels.

Interference EMG. In the second experiment, the ARV of the interference EMG during the MVC was 555.5 ± 364.0 μV at C2 and 869.2 ± 388.3 μV at C5 for the eight women. The absolute amplitude increased with increasing force (significantly different between each force level; P < 0.0001) and was significantly greater for C5 than for C2 (P < 0.05; Fig. 6A). The normalized amplitude increased with increasing force

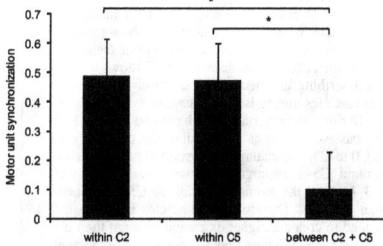

Fig. 5. Mean and SE of the synchronization of motor unit pairs within each spinal level separately and between spinal levels. The level of synchronization was similar within spinal levels but differed from the synchronization between levels. *P < 0.05.

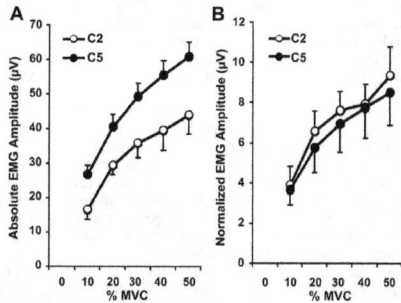

Fig. 6. Mean and SE of the absolute (A) and normalized (B) EMG amplitude detected from the semispinalis cervicis muscle at the levels of C2 and C5 during a ramped neck extension contraction from 0 to 50% MVC.

J Neurophysiol • doi:10.1152/jn.00953.2011 • www.jn.org

(significantly different between each force level; $P < 0.0001$) but was not significantly different between levels (Fig. 6*B*).

DISCUSSION

This study investigated motor unit behavior in two fascicles of the semispinalis cervicis muscle. Although there are no previous data on motor unit behavior in this muscle, the discharge rates of the studied motor units were similar to those observed in other muscles (Christou et al. 2007; Falla and Farina 2008a, 2008b; Holobar et al. 2010; Kukulka and Clamann 1981). The coefficient of variation for the interspike interval was also within the physiological range previously observed in other muscles (e.g., first dorsal interosseus, Christou et al. 2007). The main finding of the study is the difference in the strength of synaptic input delivered to different fascicles of the semispinalis cervicis muscle during constant-force extensions. This may be partly due to the different mechanical advantage of the muscle fibers in different fascicles.

The greater recruitment threshold for motor units at the C2 spinal level compared with C5 indicate that the net excitatory input to motoneurons innervating the fibers at C5 is greater than for C2 at a given force level. The greater recruitment threshold at the C2 spinal level is supported by the observation that only 18 motor units were detected at the C2 level compared with the 98 motor units detected at C5. Finally, higher absolute interference EMG amplitude was detected at C5 compared with C2 during the ramped contraction from 0 to 50% MVC, which is consistent with the observed differences in recruitment thresholds between fascicles. It must be noted, however, that absolute EMG values are not directly associated to the number of active motor units, so that EMG amplitude and number of detected units remain partly independent measures of muscle activity. First, the number of motor units detected depends on the spatial distribution of muscle fibers. Second, the amplitude of the EMG is a poor indicator of the number of detected units because of amplitude cancellation that can be very high at the analyzed contraction levels (Keenan et al. 2005). Thus a larger number of active units does not necessarily imply a proportionally greater amplitude of the EMG. Indeed, it can be proven theoretically that surface EMG amplitude is relatively insensitive to changes in motor unit activity (or motor unit number) at relatively high levels of excitation (Farina et al. 2008). For these reasons, a discrepancy between the relative difference in amplitude of the interference EMG and the relative difference in number of motor units is expected.

The preferential recruitment of motoneurons innervating fibers in specific fascicles might be explained by a nonuniform distribution of motoneuron size innervating the different fascicles, although no studies could be found in this regard. However, according to similar studies on other muscles, such as respiratory muscles (Butler and Gandevia 2008; Hudson et al. 2011), the mechanical demands of semispinalis cervicis fascicles at different spinal levels could explain a nonuniform synaptic input to motoneurons in different fascicles.

A nonuniform activation of motor units within muscle regions as found in this study has also been observed in other human muscles, such as the extensor digitorum (Keen and Fuglevand 2004), the flexor digitorum profundus (Reilly et al. 2004), the flexor digitorum superficialis (McIsaac and Fugl-

evand 2006), and the upper trapezius muscle (Falla and Farina 2008a). Furthermore, in the external intercostal muscles, a cranial-caudal (Hudson et al. 2011) and dorsal-ventral (De Troyer et al. 2003) gradient of activation has been observed. As for the semispinalis cervicis, these recruitment patterns could not be explained by a specific spatial arrangement of muscle fibers. For example, the caudal-cranial gradient for expiratory activity and the medio-lateral gradient for inspiratory activity of the internal intercostalis muscle are not due to fiber distribution, which is similar in different muscle regions (De Troyer et al. 2005). The distribution of synaptic input can diminish the influence of size in recruitment, so that other principles may be prominent. For example, motor units may be recruited according to the mechanical advantage of the muscle fibers (Butler and Gandevia 2008). This neuromechanical principle observed in inspiratory muscles appears to be preset, since it persists when all feedback possibilities are removed in experimental animals (Butler and Gandevia 2008). Similar to the observations for the intercostal muscles, different fascicles of the semispinalis cervicis muscle may be recruited to different degrees depending on the force demand for each fascicle.

Analysis of the correlation between spike trains in the time and frequency domains indicated that the input to motoneurons innervating different fascicles of the semispinalis cervicis muscle is almost independent. The low degree of synchronization between pairs of motor units detected in the present study from two individual fascicles of the semispinalis cervicis muscle indicates a different neural input to semispinalis cervicis at these levels for their independent control. This is further supported by the observation that the coherence in the 16–32 Hz band was highest for pairs of motor units from the same fascicle of the semispinalis cervicis muscle. Independent input to the two fascicles is in agreement with the observation that recruitment thresholds were significantly different for motor units at C2 and C5.

The earlier recruitment of motor units in the caudal with respect to the cranial spinal segments can be explained by different moments exerted by the fascicles of the semispinalis cervicis muscle. The force-generating capacity of a muscle can be deduced from its architectural parameters, such as physiological cross-sectional area, fascicle length, tendon length, pennation angle, and moment arm (Vasavada et al. 1998). These parameters, however, are difficult to assess for the deep cervical muscles because of their complexity (Mayoux-Benhamou et al. 1989; Vasavada et al. 1998) and, except for multifidus (Anderson et al. 2005), are largely unknown. Nevertheless, simple modeling allows a qualitative assessment of the distribution of forces for different fascicles. Figure 7 shows a schematic model describing the mechanical action of the semispinalis cervicis fascicles during isometric extension of the head. To have equilibrium, the external force has to be balanced by muscles and passive structures surrounding the cervical segments from C0 to C7. For example, the external moment to be balanced around C5–6 is larger than the external moment around C2–3, because the moment arm for the C5–6 segment is larger than at C2–3. Therefore, the fascicles spanning the joint C5–6 need to create a higher extension moment than the fascicles spanning C2–3. These conclusions are in agreement with the moment arms for extension of the different fascicles of multifidus, which decrease from ~1.4 to ~0.9 and ~0.3 cm from C6–7 to C5–6 and C4–5, respectively, for the superficial

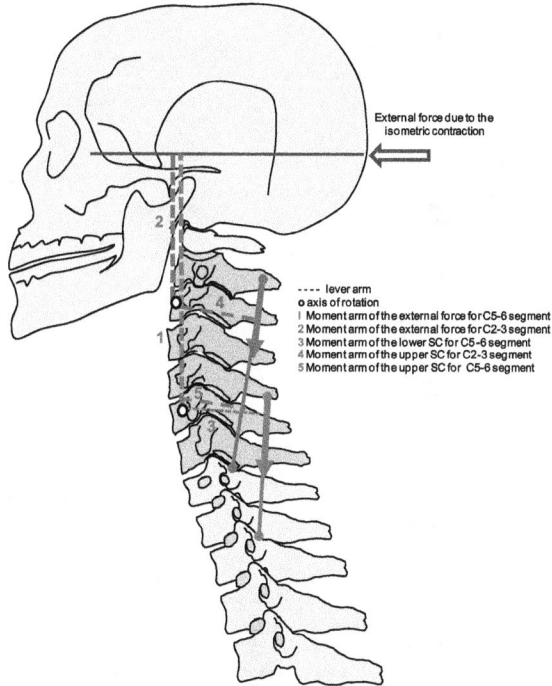

Fig. 7. Schematic representation of the moment system for the upper and lower regions of the semispinalis cervicis (SC) during isometric neck extension. The force moment of the reaction force of the head is greater for C5 than for C2. The required force to stabilize C5 is consequently higher than for C2.

External force due to the isometric contraction

---- lever arm
o axis of rotation
1 Moment arm of the external force for C5-6 segment
2 Moment arm of the external force for C2-3 segment
3 Moment arm of the lower SC for C5-6 segment
4 Moment arm of the upper SC for C2-3 segment
5 Moment arm of the upper SC for C5-6 segment

fascicles and from ~0.7 to ~0.6 and ~0.4 cm for the deep fascicles (Anderson et al. 2005).

As a limitation of this study, it must be noted that motor units were detected from only a single location within each spinal level, which, as explained above, may lead to errors in the estimation of the strength of motor unit synchronization within the fascicles. This was because of the difficulties of needle insertion medially and anterior to the fascia separating semispinalis capitis and semispinalis cervicis, in order to avoid *1*) puncture of the laterally lying arteria cervicalis profunda (Kramer et al. 2003) and *2*) penetration into the multifidus muscle, which is not always clearly separated from semispinalis cervicis by an echogenic fascia, especially at levels C2 and C5 (Kristjansson 2004; Stokes et al. 2007). Nonetheless, as discussed above, the single site insertions in each fascicle did not influence the results.

In conclusion, this study shows that individual fascicles within the semispinalis cervicis muscle are activated partly independently and with nonuniform synaptic input that allows preferential recruitment of motor units in caudal with respect to cranial fascicles.

ACKNOWLEDGMENTS

The authors are grateful to Dr. Mark de Zee, Aalborg University, for the useful discussion on the mechanical action of the semispinalis cervicis muscle.

GRANTS

This work was partly supported by the ERC Advanced Research Grant DEMOVE ("Decoding the Neural Code of Human Movements for a New Generation of Man-machine Interfaces"; no. 267888).

DISCLOSURES

No conflicts of interest, financial or otherwise, are declared by the author(s).

AUTHOR CONTRIBUTIONS

Author contributions: J.S., J.L.D., D. Farina, and D. Falla conception and design of research; J.S., J.L.D., D. Farina, and D. Falla performed experiments; J.S., J.L.D., D. Farina, and D. Falla analyzed data; J.S., J.L.D., D. Farina, and D. Falla interpreted results of experiments; J.S., J.L.D., D. Farina, and D. Falla prepared figures; J.S., J.L.D., D. Farina, and D. Falla drafted manuscript; J.S., J.L.D., D. Farina, and D. Falla edited and revised manuscript; J.S., J.L.D., D. Farina, and D. Falla approved final version of manuscript.

REFERENCES

Amjad AM, Breeze P, Conway BA, Halliday DM, Rosenberg JR. A framework for the analysis of neuronal networks. *Prog Brain Res* 80: 243–255, 1989.

Anderson JS, Hsu AW, Vasavada AN. Morphology, architecture, and biomechanics of human cervical multifidus. *Spine* 30: E86–E91, 2005.

Bergmark A. Stability of the lumbar spine. A study in mechanical engineering. *Acta Orthop Scand* 230: 1–54, 1989.

Bexander CSM, Mellor R, Hodges PW. Effect of gaze direction on neck muscle activity during cervical rotation. *Exp Brain Res* 167: 422–432, 2005.

Butler JE. Drive to the human respiratory muscles. *Respir Physiol Neurobiol* 159: 115–126, 2007.

Butler JE, Gandevia SC. The output from human inspiratory motoneurone pools. *J Physiol* 586: 1257–1264, 2008.

Christou EA, Rudroff T, Enoka JA, Meyer F, Enoka RM. Discharge rate during low-force isometric contractions influences motor unit coherence below 15 Hz but not motor unit synchronization. *Exp Brain Res* 178: 285–295, 2007.

Davey NJ, Ellaway PH, Stein RB. Statistical limits for detecting change in the cumulative sum derivative of the peristimulus time histogram. *J Neurosci Methods* 17: 153–166, 1986.

De Troyer A, Gorman RB, Gandevia SC. Distribution of inspiratory drive to the external intercostal muscles in humans. *J Physiol* 546: 943–954, 2003.

De Troyer A, Kirkwood PA, Wilson TA. Respiratory action of the intercostal muscles. *Physiol Rev* 85: 717–756, 2005.

Dideriksen JL, Falla D, Baekgaard M, Mogensen ML, Steimle KL, Farina D. Comparison between the degree of motor unit short-term synchronization and recurrence quantification analysis of the surface EMG in two human muscles. *Clin Neurophysiol* 120: 2086–2092, 2009.

Drake RL, Vogl WA, Mitchell AWM. *Gray's Anatomy.* Philadelphia, PA: Churchill Livingstone Elsevier, 2010.

Ellaway PH. Cumulative sum technique and its application to the analysis of peristimulus time histograms. *Electroencephalogr Clin Neurophysiol* 45: 302–304, 1978.

English AW, Wolf SL, Segal RL. Compartmentalization of muscles and their motor nuclei: the partitioning hypothesis. *Phys Ther* 73: 857–867, 1993.

Falla D, Farina D. Motor units in cranial and caudal regions of the upper trapezius muscle have different discharge rates during brief static contractions. *Acta Physiol (Oxf)* 192: 551–558, 2008a.

Falla D, Farina D. Non-uniform adaptation of motor unit discharge rates during sustained static contraction of the upper trapezius muscle. *Exp Brain Res* 191: 363–370, 2008b.

Falla D, Lindstrøm R, Rechter L, Farina D. Effect of pain on modulation in discharge rate of sternocleidomastoid motor units with force direction. *Clin Neurophysiol* 121: 744–753, 2010.

Farina D, Cescon C, Negro F, Enoka RM. Amplitude cancellation of motor-unit action potentials in the surface electromyogram can be estimated with spike-triggered averaging. *J Neurophysiol* 100: 431–40, 2008.

Farina D, Negro F, Gizzi L, Falla D. Low-frequency oscillations of the neural drive to the muscle are increased with experimental muscle pain. *J Neurophysiol* 107: 958–965, 2012.

Henneman E. Relation between size of neurons and their susceptibility to discharge. *Science* 126: 1345–1347, 1957.

Henneman E. The size-principle: a deterministic output emerges from a set of probabilistic connections. *J Exp Biol* 115: 105–112, 1985.

Holobar A, Minetto MA, Botter A, Negro F, Farina D. Experimental analysis of accuracy in the identification of motor unit spike trains from high-density surface EMG. *IEEE Trans Neural Syst Rehabil Eng* 18: 221–229, 2010.

Hudson AL, Gandevia SC, Butler JE. Common rostrocaudal gradient of output from human intercostal motoneurones during voluntary and automatic breathing. *Respir Physiol Neurobiol* 175: 20–28, 2011.

Hudson AL, Taylor JL, Gandevia SC, Butler JE. Coupling between mechanical and neural behaviour in the human first dorsal interosseous muscle. *J Physiol* 587: 917–926, 2009.

Keen DA, Fuglevand AJ. Common input to motor neurons innervating the same and different compartments of the human extensor digitorum muscle. *J Neurophysiol* 91: 55–62, 2004.

Keenan KG, Farina D, Maluf KS, Merletti R, Enoka RM. Influence of amplitude cancellation on the simulated surface electromyogram. *J Appl Physiol* 98: 120–131, 2005.

Kramer M, Schmid I, Sander S, Högel J, Eisele R, Kinzl L, Hartwig E. Guidelines for the intramuscular positioning of EMG electrodes in the semispinalis capitis and cervicis muscles. *J Electromyogr Kinesiol* 13: 289–295, 2003.

Kristjansson E. Reliability of ultrasonography for the cervical multifidus muscle in asymptomatic and symptomatic subjects. *Man Ther* 9: 83–88, 2004.

Kukulka CG, Clamann HP. Comparison of the recruitment and discharge properties of motor units in human brachial biceps and adductor pollicis during isometric contractions. *Brain Res* 219: 45–55, 1981.

Lee JP, Tseng WY, Shau YW, Wang CL, Wang HK, Wang SF. Measurement of segmental cervical multifidus contraction by ultrasonography in asymptomatic adults. *Man Ther* 12: 286–294, 2007.

Lord S, Barnsley L, Wallis BJ, Bogduk N. Chronic cervical zygapophysial joint pain after whiplash. *Spine* 21: 1737–1745, 1996.

Mayoux-Benhamou MA, Wybier M, Revel M. Strength and cross-sectional area of the dorsal neck muscles. *Ergonomics* 32: 513–518, 1989.

McGill KC, Lateva ZC, Marateb HR. EMGLAB: an interactive EMG decomposition program. *J Neurosci Methods* 149: 121–133, 2005.

McIsaac TL, Fuglevand AJ. Motor-unit synchrony within and across compartments of the human flexor digitorum superficialis. *J Neurophysiol* 97: 550–556, 2006.

Nordstrom MA, Fuglevand AJ, Enoka RM. Estimating the strength of common input to human motoneurons from the cross-correlogram. *J Physiol* 453: 547–574, 1992.

Reilly KT, Nordstrom MA, Schieber MH. Short-term synchronization between motor units in different functional subdivisions of the human flexor digitorum profundus muscle. *J Neurophysiol* 92: 734–742, 2004.

Rosenberg JR, Amjad AM, Breeze P, Brillinger DR, Halliday DM. The Fourier approach to the identification of functional coupling between neuronal spike trains. *Prog Biophys Mol Biol* 53: 1–31, 1989.

Schuenke M, Schulte E, Schumacher U. *Thieme Atlas of Anatomy, General Anatomy and Musculoskeletal System.* Stuttgart, Germany: Thieme, 2006.

Semmler JG, Nordstrom MA, Wallace CJ. Relationship between motor unit short-term synchronization and common drive in human first dorsal interosseous muscle. *Brain Res* 767: 314–320, 1997.

Stokes M, Hides J, Elliott JM, Kiesel K, Hodges PW. Rehabilitative ultrasound imaging of the posterior paraspinal muscles. *J Orthop Sports Phys Ther* 37: 581–595, 2007.

ter Haar Romeny BM, Denier van der Gon JJ, Gielen CC. Changes in recruitment order of motor units in the human biceps muscle. *Exp Neurol* 78: 360–368, 1982.

ter Haar Romeny BM, van der Gon JJ, and Gielen CC. Relation between location of a motor unit in the human biceps brachii and its critical firing levels for different tasks. *Exp Neurol* 85: 631–650, 1984.

Vasavada AN, Siping L, Scott D. Influence of muscle morphometry and moment arms on the moment-generating capacity of human neck muscles. *Spine* 23: 412–422, 1998.

Whittaker JL, Teyhen DS, Elliott JM, Cook K, Langevin HM, Dahl HH, Stokes M. Rehabilitative ultrasound imaging: understanding the technology and its applications. *J Orthop Sports Phys Ther* 37: 434–449, 2007.

Clinical Neurophysiology 123 (2012) 1403–1408

Contents lists available at SciVerse ScienceDirect

Clinical Neurophysiology

journal homepage: www.elsevier.com/locate/clinph

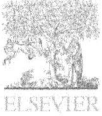

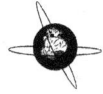

Chronic trauma-induced neck pain impairs the neural control of the deep semispinalis cervicis muscle

Jochen Schomacher[a], Dario Farina[b], René Lindstroem[a], Deborah Falla[b,c,*]

[a] Center for Sensory-Motor Interaction (SMI), Department of Health Science and Technology, Aalborg University, Denmark
[b] Department of Neurorehabilitation Engineering, Bernstein Focus Neurotechnology (BFNT) Göttingen, Bernstein Center for Computational Neuroscience, University Medical Center Göttingen, Georg-August University, Göttingen, Germany
[c] Pain Clinic, Center for Anesthesiology, Emergency and Intensive Care Medicine, University Hospital Göttingen, Göttingen, Germany

ARTICLE INFO

Article history:
Accepted 25 November 2011
Available online 27 December 2011

Keywords:
Neck pain
Semispinalis cervicis
EMG
Tuning curves

HIGHLIGHTS

- This study is the first to present neurophysiological data from the deep semispinalis cervicis muscle in patients with chronic neck pain.
- Patients with neck pain showed reduced and less defined activity of the semispinalis cervicis muscle during a multidirectional isometric task.
- This finding might be relevant for the maintenance or recurrence of neck pain.

ABSTRACT

Objective: The deep cervical extensors show structural changes in patients with neck pain however their activation has never been investigated in patients. This study is the first to present neurophysiological data from the deep semispinalis cervicis muscle in patients.

Methods: Ten women with chronic neck pain and 10 healthy controls participated. Activity of the semispinalis cervicis was measured as subjects performed isometric contractions at 15 and 30 N force with continuous change in force direction in the range 0–360°. Tuning curves of the EMG amplitude (average rectified value, ARV) were computed and the mean point of the ARV curves defined a directional vector, which determined the directional specificity of the muscle activity.

Results: Patients displayed reduced directional specificity of the semispinalis cervicis ($P < 0.05$). Furthermore, the EMG amplitude during the circular contraction was lower for the patients (86.3 ± 38.0 and 104.4 ± 47.0 μV for 15 and 30 N, respectively) compared to controls (226.4 ± 128.5 and 315.8 ± 205.5 μV; $P < 0.05$).

Conclusions: The activity of the semispinalis cervicis muscle is reduced and less defined in patients with neck pain confirming a disturbance in the neural control of this muscle.

Significance: This finding suggests that exercises that target the deep semispinalis cervicis muscle may be relevant to include in the management of patients with neck pain.

© 2011 International Federation of Clinical Neurophysiology. Published by Elsevier Ireland Ltd. All rights reserved.

1. Introduction

The neck extensors are organized in four layers (Stokes et al., 2007). Levator scapulae and upper trapezius constitute the superficial layer and, although they have attachments to the cranium and cervical spine, they are primarily considered muscles of the shoulder girdle (Mayoux-Benhamou et al., 1997). Splenius capitis constitutes the next layer and acts on the head to produce extension, ipsilateral rotation and ipsilateral side bending of the neck (Sommerich et al., 2000). The semispinalis capitis and semispinalis cervicis form the third layer (Conley et al., 1997; Vasavada et al., 1998) although most often the semispinalis cervicis is considered together with the multifidus and rotatores muscles as the deepest layer of the cervical extensors (Blouin et al., 2007; Rankin et al., 2005; Stokes et al., 2007) together with the deep cranio-cervical muscles; the rectus capitis posterior major and minor, and obliquus capitis inferior and superior. The semispinalis cervicis has the same osseous insertions as multifidus (Mayoux-Benhamou et al., 1997) and together they are considered key muscles for cervical spine segmental support due to their relatively small moment arms, attachments to adjacent vertebrae (Blouin et al., 2007) and high proportion (~70%) of slow twitch fibres (Boyd-Clark et al., 2001).

* Corresponding author at: Pain Clinic, Center for Anesthesiology, Emergency and Intensive Care Medicine, University Hospital Göttingen, Robert-Koch-Str. 40, 37075 Göttingen, Germany. Tel.: +49 (0) 551 3920109; fax: + 49 (0) 551 3920110.
E-mail address: deborah.falla@bccn.uni-goettingen.de (D. Falla).

1388-2457/$36.00 © 2011 International Federation of Clinical Neurophysiology. Published by Elsevier Ireland Ltd. All rights reserved.
doi:10.1016/j.clinph.2011.11.033

Ultrasound and magnetic resonance imaging studies have shown alterations in the physical characteristics of the cervical extensors in patients with whiplash-induced neck pain including reduced cross-sectional area (CSA) of the multifidus and semispinalis cervicis muscles (Kristjansson, 2004; Elliott et al., 2008b) and fatty infiltrate of the deep and superficial extensors (Elliott et al., 2006). In addition, studies have reported reduced CSA of the multifidus (Fernández-de-las-Peñas et al., 2008) and semispinalis capitis muscle (Rezasoltani et al., 2010) in patients with non-traumatic neck pain. Structural changes in the deep neck extensor muscles have been attributed to factors such as generalized disuse (Elliott et al., 2006), chronic denervation (Andary et al., 1998), functional adaptation in response to altered activity in other muscles (Elliott et al., 2008b), facet joint trauma (Elliott et al., 2006, 2008b) or involvement of the sympathetic nervous system (Passatore and Roatta, 2006; Roatta et al., 2008). Regardless of the mechanism underlying these observations, changes in the physical properties of the deep neck extensor muscles may lead to compromised function of the cervical spine. However, to date there has been very few neurophysiological studies investigating the activation of the deep neck extensors and those that have been performed have been limited to individuals without known impairment or pathology (Mayoux-Benhamou et al., 1997; Blouin et al., 2007). Thus the purpose of this study was to compare the activation of the semispinalis cervicis muscle during a multidirectional isometric task between patients with chronic neck pain and healthy controls.

2. Methods

2.1. Subjects

Ten women (age, mean ± SD: 30.4 ± 7.0 years; height: 167.5 ± 5.3 cm; weight: 60.7 ± 10.7 kg) with chronic, trauma-induced neck pain participated in the study. Their average duration of pain was 5.7 ± 1.6 years (range: 3.1–7.5 years). Six of the women had pain induced by a motor vehicle accident and four from a fall. Trauma-induced neck pain was chosen since structural changes of the cervical extensor muscles have been frequently observed in this patient group (Elliott et al., 2008a). To be included patients had to be aged between 18 and 45 years and rate their pain intensity (average over the last week) greater than 3 on a 10 cm visual analogue scale (VAS). Patients were excluded if they had undergone cervical spine surgery, reported any neurological sign, had participated in a neck exercise program in the past 12 months, or were undergoing treatment at the time of testing. The patients' average score for the Neck Disability Index (0–50) (Vernon and Mior, 1991) was 21.2 ± 5.7 (range: 11–32) and their average pain intensity rated on a VAS (0–10) was 5.8 ± 1.6 (range: 3.1–8.0).

Ten healthy women (age, mean ± SD: 26.8 ± 5.9 years; height: 168.3 ± 7.0 cm; weight: 63.3 ± 10.5 kg) were recruited as controls. Control subjects were included if they were free of neck pain, had not had neck surgery and had no history of neurological disorders. Ethical approval for the study was granted by the Regional Ethics Committee (N-20090039). All participants provided written informed consent and procedures were conducted according to the Declaration of Helsinki.

2.2. Electromyography

Intramuscular EMG was acquired from the semispinalis cervicis muscle at the level of the 3rd spinous process (C3) unilaterally. Control subjects were measured on the right side, whereas patients were measured on the side of greatest pain (right side for eight patients). Wire electrodes made of Teflon-coated stainless steel

(diameter: 0.1 mm; A–M Systems, Carlsborg, WA) were inserted into the muscle via a 27-gauge hypodermic needle. Approximately 3–4 mm of insulation was removed from the tip of the wires to obtain an interference EMG signal. Needle insertion (Fig. 1) was guided by ultrasound (Acuson 128 Computed Sonography, Canada) using a 10-MHz linear transducer (Bexander et al., 2005; Lee et al., 2007). Ultrasound is a reliable tool to visualize the deep neck extensors (Kristjansson, 2004; Stokes et al., 2007).

Participants were positioned in prone with their head in a neutral position. The spinous process of the second cervical vertebrae was located by palpation as the first bony landmark caudal to the occiput and a cutaneous landmark was made at the level of the third cervical spinous process (Lee et al., 2007). The ultrasound transducer was placed transversally in the midline over C3 and moved laterally to image the extensor muscles. The identification of the echogenic (bright and reflective) laminae and the spinous processes are the main bony landmarks for identifying the cervical extensors which are separated by echogenic fascia layers (Stokes et al., 2007). The fascia between the semispinalis cervicis and multifidus muscle is often difficult to distinguish (Kristjansson, 2004). However, the fascia between the semispinalis capitis and semispinalis cervicis is clearly visible (Kramer et al., 2003) thus the needle was inserted just below this fascia. The insertion point of the needle was 1.5 cm lateral to the midline and the needle was inserted vertically as previously described (Kramer et al., 2003). Following skin preparation (injection swabs: 70% isopropylalkohol, 30 × 30 mm, Selefatrade, Spånga, Sweden), the needle containing the wire was inserted into the muscle belly and the needle removed immediately leaving the wire in the muscle for the duration of the experiment.

Signals were acquired in monopolar mode. A reference electrode was placed around the wrist. EMG signals were amplified (EMG-USB2, 256-channel EMG amplifier, LISiN-OT Bioelettronica, Torino, Italy; 500 Hz–5 kHz), sampled at 10,000 Hz, and converted to digital form by a 12-bit analog-to-digital converter.

2.3. Procedure

The participants were seated with their head rigidly fixed in a device for the measurement of multidirectional neck force with their back supported, knees and hips in 90° of flexion, their torso firmly strapped to the seat back and their hands resting comfortably on their lap (Falla et al., 2010). The device is equipped with eight adjustable contacts which are fastened around the head to stabilize the head and provide resistance during isometric contractions of the neck. The force device is equipped with force transducers (strain gauges) to measure force in the sagittal and coronal planes. The electrical signals from the strain gauges were amplified (LISiN–OT Bioelettronica, Torino, Italy) and their output was displayed on an oscilloscope as visual feedback to the subject.

Following a period of familiarization with the measuring device and a period to practice the desired contractions, subjects performed two neck extension maximum voluntary contractions (MVC) separated by 1 min of rest. Verbal encouragement was provided to the subject. The highest value of force recorded over the two maximum contractions was selected as the maximal force.

A rest of ~5 min followed the MVCs. Subsequently, the subjects performed contractions in the horizontal plane at 15 and 30 N force with change in force direction in the range 0–360° (circular contractions; 0°: flexion, 90° right lateral flexion, 180° extension, 270° left lateral flexion). Real-time visual feedback of force direction and magnitude was provided on an oscilloscope positioned in front of the subject. A 15 or 30 N circle template was superimposed on the oscilloscope to guide the subjects. Following a period of ~10 min to practice the task, the subjects performed the 15 and 30 N contractions in both clockwise and counter-clockwise

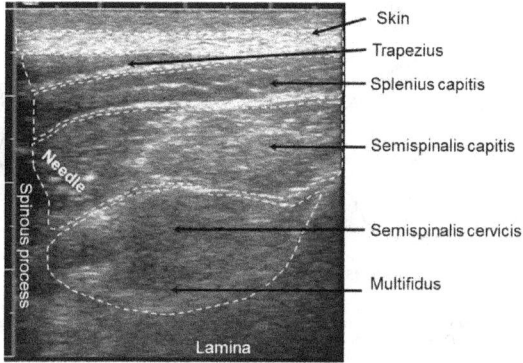

Fig. 1. Ultrasound image of the neck extensors taken at the level of the third cervical vertebrae (right side) with the needle insertion into the semispinalis cervicis muscle.

directions with 2-min of rest between contractions. The subjects were guided by a counter to perform the circular contractions at a constant velocity in 12-s.

2.4. Signal analysis

During the circular contractions, the amplitude of the intramuscular EMG was estimated as the average rectified value (ARV) of the signal in non-overlapping intervals of 250 ms. The ARV of the EMG as a function of the angle of force direction will be referred to in the following as directional activation curves. The directional activation curves represent the modulation in intensity of muscle activity with the direction of force exertion and represent a closed area when expressed in polar coordinates. The line connecting the origin with the central point of this area defined a directional vector, whose length was expressed as a percent of the mean ARV during the entire task. This normalized vector length represents the specificity of muscle activation: it is equal to zero if the muscle is active in the same way in all directions and, conversely, it corresponds to 100% if the muscle is active in exclusively one direction. In addition, the EMG amplitude was averaged across the entire circular contraction to provide an indicator of the overall muscle activity. Since no significant differences were observed for the data extracted from the circular contractions in the clockwise and counter-clockwise directions when the data were compared for the same direction of force, the data were combined to obtain an average.

The coefficient of variation of force (SD divided by mean, %) was also obtained for the circular contractions.

2.5. Statistical analysis

A one-way analysis of variance (ANOVA) was used to evaluate differences between patients and controls for maximum neck extension strength with group (patient and control) as the between subjects variable. Two-way ANOVAs were used to assess differences in the directional specificity of muscle activity (vector length), mean activity and coefficient of variation of force with force (15 and 30 N) as the within subject variable and group (patient and control) as the between subject variable. Significant differences revealed by ANOVA were followed by post hoc Student–Newman–Keuls (SNK) pair-wise comparisons. Results are reported as mean and SD in the text and SE in the figures. Statistical significance was set at $P < 0.05$.

3. Results

Patients displayed significantly reduced maximum neck extension force compared to controls (125.7 ± 55.2 and 209.2 ± 56.9 N, respectively; $P < 0.01$).

Fig. 2 shows representative force traces during a circular contraction performed at 15 N in the counter-clockwise direction for a control subject and a patient. In this example, the patient presents with less accuracy in producing the circular contraction compared to the control subject. From the group data analysis, the patients presented with a greater coefficient of variation of force compared to the control group during the circular contractions both at 15 and 30 N (average; controls: $11.8 \pm 1.7\%$, patients: $14.8 \pm 4.9\%$; $F = 4.9$; $P < 0.05$).

Fig. 3 presents the force and intramuscular EMG signals during a 15 N circular contraction performed in the counter-clockwise direction by representative subjects in the two groups. In this example, the patient shows an intramuscular EMG signal with similar amplitude, and overall lower EMG amplitude in all force directions. Conversely, the control subject displays a more steady maintenance of force and a greater modulation in the activity of the semispinalis cervicis muscle with force direction.

The mean activity of the semispinalis cervicis (averaged across the circular contractions) was greater for the 30 N contraction compared to the 15 N for both patients and controls ($F = 14.4$; $P < 0.01$). However, the activity of semispinalis cervicis was lower for the patients for both the 15 and 30 N contractions ($F = 10.5$; $P < 0.01$) compared to the control subjects (Fig. 4).

Representative directional activation curves during a circular contraction performed at 15 and 30 N are illustrated in Fig. 5 for a control subject and a patient. In this example, the control subject presents with defined activation of the semispinalis cervicis with the highest amplitude of activity towards ipsilateral posterolateral extension. Conversely, the directional activation curve for the representative patient indicates more even activation levels of the semispinalis cervicis muscle for all directions.

Values of directional specificity in the EMG of the semispinalis cervicis muscle increased with load (average across groups: $23.0 \pm 9.8\%$ and $28.9 \pm 10.4\%$ for the 15 and 30 N contractions respectively; $F = 5.2$; $P < 0.05$). However, as observed in Fig. 6, the directional specificity was reduced in the patient group for both the 15 and 30 N circular contractions ($F = 4.7$; $P < 0.05$).

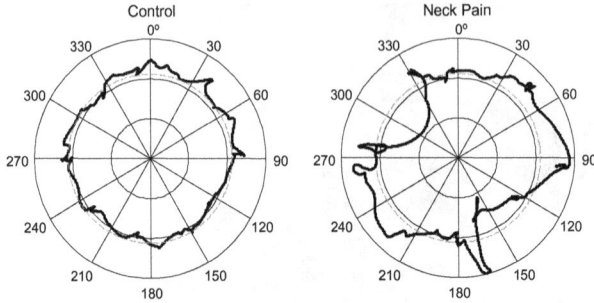

Fig. 2. Representative force traces obtained for a control subject and a patient performing a circular contraction at 15 N in the counter-clockwise direction. In this example the coefficient of variation of force is 7.4% and 17.5% for the control and patient respectively.

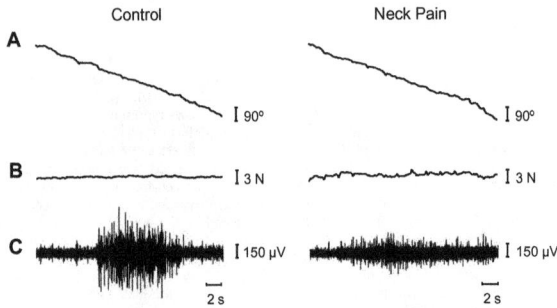

Fig. 3. Representative angle (A), force (B) and (C) intramuscular EMG data acquired from the semispinalis cervicis muscle of one control subject and one patient during a 15 N circular contraction performed in the counter-clockwise direction. Note the reduced force steadiness and similar EMG amplitude in all force directions for the patient.

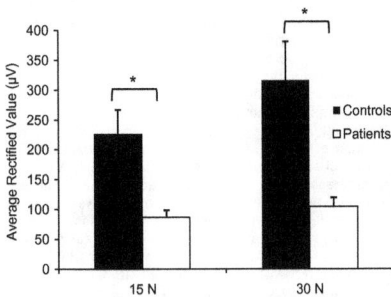

Fig. 4. Mean and standard deviation of the average rectified value of the intramuscular EMG of semispinalis cervicis muscle obtained during the circular contractions at both 15 and 30 N of force for the control subjects and patients with neck pain. *$P < 0.001$.

4. Discussion

This study examined the activation of the deep semispinalis cervicis muscle in patients with trauma-induced chronic neck pain. The results showed that, contrary to asymptomatic individuals, the semispinalis cervicis muscle has reduced and less defined activity during a multidirectional isometric contraction in patients with chronic neck pain. Reduced activation of the semispinalis cervicis may impact on support of the cervical spine which could be relevant for the maintenance and perpetuation of neck pain.

For the control subjects the activity of the semispinalis cervicis muscle was tuned selectively for the direction of force, i.e. the muscle was active predominately in extension with a small ipsilateral component. This is in agreement with other studies on asymptomatic subjects showing well-defined preferred directions of activation of the neck muscles (Blouin et al., 2007; Falla et al., 2010; Lindstrøm et al., 2011). The preferred direction of activity observed for the semispinalis cervicis confirms its role as a primary extensor (Conley et al., 1997). The increased directional specificity of semispinalis cervicis activity at 30 N compared to 15 N also confirms observations for other neck muscles, such as the sternocleidomastoid, semispinalis capitis, splenius capitis and upper trapezius,

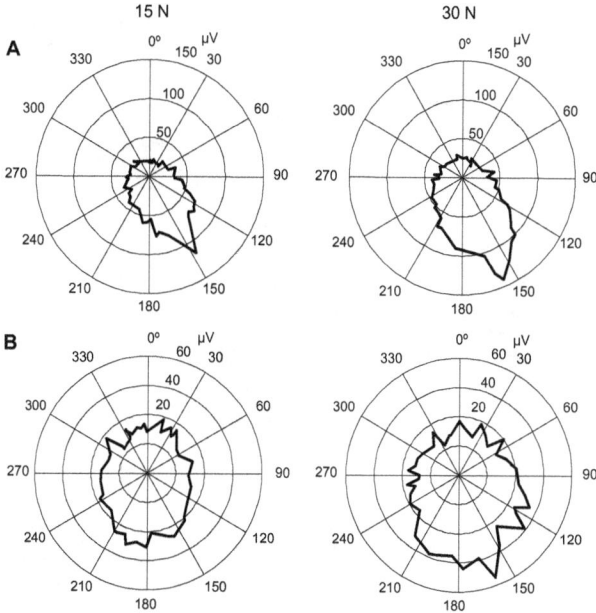

Fig. 5. Representative directional activation curves for a control subject (A) and a patient (B) performing circular contractions at 15 and 30 N of force.

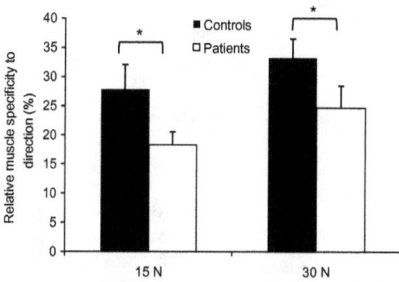

Fig. 6. Mean and standard deviation of the directional specificity in the intramuscular EMG of the semispinalis cervicis muscle obtained during the circular contractions at both 15 and 30 N of force for the control subjects and patients with neck pain. *P < 0.05.

suggesting that at lower loads multiple muscles can be recruited to generate the required load in a desired direction, while at higher loads the primary muscles are predominately recruited (Blouin et al., 2007).

In contrast to the control subjects, the patient group showed reduced specificity of semispinalis cervicis activity. Reduced specificity of activity has also been observed for both the sternocleidomastoid and splenius capitis muscles in patients with neck pain

which is largely due to increased activation of the muscle when acting as an antagonist (Falla et al., 2010; Lindstrøm et al., 2011). However reduced specificity of both the sternocleidomastoid and splenius capitis was associated with an overall increase in activity in patients with neck pain (Falla et al., 2010; Lindstrøm et al., 2011). The opposite was observed for the semispinalis cervicis muscle in this study. Despite reduced specificity of activity and increased coactivation, the muscle displayed reduced activity overall in the patient group. This finding is in accordance with observations from the deep cervical flexor muscles, the longus colli and longus capitis, which also show reduced activity in patients with chronic neck pain (Falla et al., 2004).

Studies examining the structure of the deep neck extensors in patients with whiplash-induced neck pain show both fatty infiltration (Elliott et al., 2006) and atrophy of the semispinalis cervicis (Elliott et al., 2008b) and multifidus muscle (Kristjansson, 2004). Atrophy of the multifidus (Fernández-de-las-Peñas et al., 2008) and semispinalis capitis muscle (Rezasoltani et al., 2010) has also been observed in patients with idiopathic neck pain. The findings in this study confirm the dysfunction of the deep neck extensor muscles by demonstrating reduced neural drive to the semispinalis cervicis muscle in patients with chronic trauma-induced neck pain. Reduced activation of the deep neck muscles, including the semispinalis cervicis, may be attributed to a number of mechanisms. The pain adaptation model describes an inhibition of agonist muscles with a simultaneous increase of antagonist activity in order to limit the range and velocity of motion (Lund et al., 1991). This theory is supported by several experimental studies (Graven-Nielsen et al., 1997; Birch et al., 2000). However, as recently discussed, the pain adaptation model is not always consistent with clinical observations (Türker, 2010).

Previous studies suggest that the central motor strategy is different in the presence of neck pain. When pain is acutely induced in the neck muscles of healthy subjects, the coordination among neck muscles is substantially altered (Falla et al., 2007). Previous clinical data also show the presence of altered motor strategies suggestive of changes in motor planning. For example, onset of the deep cervical flexors (longus colli and longus capitis) is delayed in chronic neck pain patients and is not a preplanned response compared to healthy controls (Falla et al., 2004). Thus, the reduced activation of the deep semispinalis cervicis muscle in the patient group may be attributed to an altered motor strategy for the task.

4.1. Methodological considerations

The main limitation of the study is the small sample size. This was necessary due to the invasiveness of the procedure. Despite the small sample, the findings were consistent across subjects and yielded significant results.

4.2. Clinical considerations

Static and dynamic control of the head and neck is provided by multiple muscles surrounding the cervical spine. Muscles are arranged in separate layers and due to their morphological differences they provide distinct mechanical effects on the spine. Semispinalis cervicis, together with multifidus, forms the transversospinalis muscle (Anderson et al., 2005) which contributes to segmental support by attaching directly to the vertebrae (Sommerich et al., 2000; Blouin et al., 2007). This function cannot be replicated by the more superficial muscles and is based on the anatomical characteristics (Blouin et al., 2007) and histological composition (Boyd-Clark et al., 2001) of the muscle.

Potentially, reduced activation of the semispinalis cervicis muscle may compromise cervical spine stability increasing the risk of micro-/macro-trauma which can perpetuate and maintain neck pain (Pearson et al., 2004; Bogduk and McGuirk, 2006). The finding of reduced activation of the semispinalis cervicis in patients with neck pain supports the prescription of specific exercises to retrain the deep extensors in patients with neck pain (Jull et al., 2008; Elliott et al., 2010).

5. Conclusion

This study provides evidence of altered activation of the semispinalis cervicis muscle in patients with neck pain. This finding may have implications for the recurrence of neck pain and suggests that exercises that target the deep neck extensors may be relevant to include in the management of patients with neck pain.

Acknowledgements

The authors declare no conflict of interest.

References

Andary MT, Hallgren RC, Greenman PE, Rechtien JJ. Neurogenic atrophy of suboccipital muscles after a cervical injury: a case study. Am J Phys Med Rehabil 1998;77:545–9.
Anderson JS, Hsu AW, Vasavada AN. Morphology, architecture, and biomechanics of human cervical multifidus. Spine 2005;30:E86–91.
Bexander CSM, Mellor R, Hodges PW. Effect of gaze direction on neck muscle activity during cervical rotation. Exp Brain Res 2005;167:422–32.
Birch L, Christensen H, Arendt-Nielsen L, Graven-Nielsen T, Søgaard K. The influence of experimental muscle pain on motor unit activity during low-level contraction. European J Appl Physiol 2000;83:200–6.
Blouin J-S, Siegmund GP, Carpenter MG, Inglis JT. Neural control of superficial and deep neck muscles in humans. J Neurophysiol 2007;98:920–8.
Bogduk N, McGuirk B. Management of acute and chronic neck pain, an evidence-based approach. Edinburgh: Elsevier; 2006.
Boyd-Clark LC, Briggs CA, Galea MP. Comparative histochemical composition of muscle fibres in a pre- and postvertebral muscle of the cervical spine. J Anat 2001;199:709–16.
Conley MS, Stone MH, Nimmons M, Dudley GA. Resistance training and human cervical muscle recruitment plasticity. J Appl Physiol 1997;83:2105–11.
Elliott J, Sterling M, Noteboom JT, Darnell R, Galloway G, Jull G. Fatty infiltrate in the cervical extensor muscles is not a feature of chronic, insidious-onset neck pain. Clin Radiol 2008a;63:681–7.
Elliott JM, Jull G, Noteboom JT, Darnell R, Galloway G, Gibbon WW. Fatty infiltration in the cervical extensor muscles in persistent whiplash-associated disorders: a magnetic resonance imaging analysis. Spine 2006;31:E847–55.
Elliott JM, Jull G, Noteboom JT, Galloway G. MRI study of the cross-sectional area for the cervical extensor musculature in patients with persistent whiplash associated disorders (WAD). Man Ther 2008b;13:258–65.
Elliott JM, O'Leary SP, Cagnie B, Durbridge G, Danneels L, Jull G. Craniocervical orientation affects muscle activation when exercising the cervical extensors in healthy subjects. Arch Phys Med Rehabil 2010;91:1418–22.
Falla D, Farina D, Dahl MK, Graven-Nielsen T. Muscle pain induces task-dependent changes in cervical agonist/antagonist activity. J Appl Physiol 2007;102:601–9.
Falla D, Jull G, Hodges PW. Feedforward activity of the cervical flexor muscles during voluntary arm movements is delayed in chronic neck pain. Exp Brain Res 2004;157:43–8.
Falla D, Lindstrøm R, Rechter L, Farina D. Effect of pain on modulation in discharge rate of sternocleidomastoid motor units with force direction. Clin Neurophysiol 2010;121:744–53.
Fernández-de-las-Peñas C, Albert-Sanchís JC, Buil M, Benitez JC, Alburquerque-Sendín F. Cross-sectional area of cervical multifidus muscle in females with chronic bilateral neck pain compared to controls. J Orthop Sports Physical Therapy 2008;38:175–80.
Graven-Nielsen T, Svensson P, Arendt-Nielsen L. Effects of experimental muscle pain on muscle activity and co-ordination during static and dynamic motor function. Electroencephalogr Clin Neurophysiol 1997;10:156–64.
Jull G, Sterling M, Falla D, Treleaven J, O'Leary S. Whiplash, headache, and neck pain: research-based directions for physical therapies: research-based directions for physical therapies. Edinburgh: Churchill Livingstone (Elsevier); 2008.
Kramer M, Schmid I, Sander S, Högel J, Eisele R, Kinzl L, et al. Guidelines for the intramuscular positioning of EMG electrodes in the semispinalis capitis and cervicis muscles. J Electromyogr Kinesiol 2003;13:289–95.
Kristjansson E. Reliability of ultrasonography for the cervical multifidus muscle in asymptomatic and symptomatic subjects. Man Ther 2004;9:83–8.
Lee JP, Tseng WY, Shau YW, Wang CL, Wang HK, Wang SF. Measurement of segmental cervical multifidus contraction by ultrasonography in asymptomatic adults. Man Ther 2007;12:286–94.
Lindstrøm R, Schomacher J, Farina D, Rechter L, Falla D. Association between neck muscle coactivation, pain, and strength in women with neck pain. Man Ther 2011;16:80–6.
Lund JP, Donga R, Widmer CG, Stohler CS. The pain-adaptation model: a discussion of the relationship between musculoskeletal pain and motor activity. Can J Physiol Pharmacol 1991;49:683–94.
Mayoux-Benhamou MA, Revel M, Vallee C. Selective electromyography of dorsal neck muscles in humans. Exp Brain Res 1997;113:353–60.
Passatore M, Roatta S. Influence of sympathetic nervous system on sensorimotor function: whiplash associated disorders (WAD) as a model. Eur J Appl Physiol 2006;98:423–49.
Pearson AM, Ivanicic PC, Ito S, Panjabi MM. Facet joint kinematics and injury mechanisms during simulated whiplash. Spine 2004;29:390–7.
Rankin G, Stokes M, Newham DJ. Size and shape of the posterior neck muscles measured by ultrasound imaging: normal values in males and females of different ages. Man Ther 2005;10:108–15.
Rezasoltani A, Ali-Reza A, Khosro K-K, Abbass R. Preliminary study of neck muscle size and strength measurements in females with chronic non-specific neck pain and healthy control subjects. Man Ther 2010;15:400–3.
Roatta S, Arendt-Nielsen L, Farina D. Sympathetic-induced changes in discharge rate and spike-triggered average twitch torque of low-threshold motor units in humans. J Physiol 2008;586:5561–74.
Sommerich CM, Joines SMB, Hermans V, Moon SD. Use of surface electromyography to estimate neck muscle activity. J Electromyogr Kinesiol 2000;10:377–98.
Stokes M, Hides J, Elliott JM, Kiesel K, Hodges PW. Rehabilitative ultrasound imaging of the posterior paraspinal muscles. J Orthop Sports Phys Ther 2007;37:581–95.
Türker KS. Muscle pain theories: is there a third dimension? Clin Neurophysiol 2010;121:634–5.
Vasavada AN, Siping L, Scott D. Influence of muscle morphometry and moment arms on the moment-generating capacity of human neck muscles. Spine 1998;23:412–22.
Vernon H, Mior S. The neck disability index: a study of reliability and validity. J Manipulative Physiol Ther 1991;14:409–15.

Localized Pressure Pain Sensitivity is Associated With Lower Activation of the Semispinalis Cervicis Muscle in Patients With Chronic Neck Pain

Jochen Schomacher, MSc, Shellie A. Boudreau, PhD,* Frank Petzke, PD, Dr med,†
and Deborah Falla, PhD†‡*

Objective: To investigate the relation between localized pressure pain sensitivity and the amplitude and specificity of semispinalis cervicis muscle activity in patients with chronic neck pain.

Materials and Methods: Pressure pain detection thresholds (PPDTs) were measured over the C2-C3 and C5-C6 cervical zygapophyseal joints in 10 women with chronic neck pain and 9 healthy age-matched and sex-matched controls. Intramuscular electromyography (EMG) was acquired from the semispinalis cervicis at the levels of C2 and C5 during isometric circular contractions in the horizontal plane at 15 and 30 N, with continuous change in force direction in the range 0 to 360 degrees. The average rectified value and directional specificity of semispinalis cervicis muscle activity were computed and regression analyses were performed between measures of EMG and PPDT.

Results: Patients showed significantly lower PPDT compared with controls ($P < 0.01$). Patients also displayed lower EMG amplitude of the semispinalis cervicis at both spinal levels during the circular contractions (average across spinal levels, mean ± SD: 129.01 ± 58.99 and 126.83 ± 58.78 μV for the 15- and 30-N contractions, respectively) compared with controls (158.69 ± 66.27 and 187.64 ± 87.82 μV; $P < 0.05$). Furthermore, the directional specificity of semispinalis cervicis muscle was lower for the patients during the circular contractions ($P < 0.05$). The PPDT (C2 and C5 pooled) was positively correlated to both, directional specificity ($R^2 = 0.22$, $P < 0.05$) and amplitude ($R^2 = 0.15$, $P < 0.05$) of the EMG.

Discussion: In contrast to asymptomatic individuals, the semispinalis cervicis muscle displays reduced and less-defined EMG activity during a multidirectional isometric contraction in patients with chronic neck pain. The altered behavior of the semispinalis cervicis is weakly associated to pressure pain sensitivity.

Key Words: pressure pain detection thresholds, semispinalis cervicis, neck pain, EMG

(Clin J Pain 2013;00:000–000)

Received for publication June 8, 2012; accepted October 11, 2012.
From the *Department of Health Science and Technology, Center for Sensory-Motor Interaction (SMI), Aalborg University, Aalborg, Denmark; †Pain Clinic, Center for Anesthesiology, Emergency and Intensive Care Medicine, University Hospital Göttingen; and ‡Department of Neurorehabilitation Engineering, Bernstein Focus Neurotechnology (BFNT) Göttingen, Bernstein Center for Computational Neuroscience, University Medical Center Göttingen, Georg-August University, Göttingen, Germany.
The authors declare no conflict of interest. No funding was received by the National Institutes of Health (NIH), MD, Wellcome Trust, London UK, Howard Hughes Medical Institute (HHMI) MD, or others.
Reprints: Deborah Falla, PhD, Pain Clinic, Center for Anesthesiology, Emergency and Intensive Care Medicine, University Hospital Göttingen, Robert-Koch-Str 40, Göttingen 37075, Germany (e-mail: deborah.falla@bccn.uni-goettingen.de).
Copyright © 2013 by Lippincott Williams & Wilkins

N umerous studies have demonstrated that neck pain is associated with altered behavior of the cervical muscles.[1–6] In particular, the deep cervical muscles show dysfunction in patients with chronic neck pain (CNP) including reduced activation of the deep cervical flexors during a task of craniocervical flexion[7] and lower activation of the deep semispinalis cervicis muscle during multidirectional isometric contractions,[8] and during cervical extension performed in a neutral craniocervical position.[9] Furthermore, the semispinalis cervicis muscle shows lower directional specificity of activation in patients with CNP, that is, patients demonstrate a reduced ability to produce a well-defined muscular activation that appropriately reflects the anatomic position of the semispinalis cervicis relative to the spine during the performance of circular isometric contractions.[8]

The mechanisms underlying lower activation of the deep cervical muscles in patients with neck pain remain unclear and the variability of change in muscle activation observed across patients is not fully understood. There is some evidence that the variability of neck muscle activation is related to the magnitude of pain and thus the individual variability of patient presentation. For example, higher levels of pain were associated with greater delays in the activation of the deep cervical flexors during rapid flexion of the shoulder and lower amplitude of activation during isometric craniocervical flexion contractions.[10] This data partially support the pain adaptation model.[11] This theory is also supported by several experimental studies.[12,13] However, as discussed recently, the pain adaptation model is not always consistent with clinical observations as the adaptation to pain appears dependent on the muscle and task investigated.[14–16]

It is unknown, however, whether hyperalgesia on palpation of the cervical spine is correlated to lower amplitude and lower directional specificity of deep cervical extensor muscle activity. Hyperalgesia is common in patients with CNP and can be measured by the pressure pain detection threshold (PPDT).[17] The assessment of the PPDT is commonly applied over the cervical structures to assess the effect of exercise on CNP,[18] to predict short-term neck-related disability scores,[19] and to describe or categorize patients with neck pain.[20] Therefore, the purpose of this study was to investigate the relationship between localized pressure pain sensitivity over cervical zygapophyseal joints and the amplitude and specificity of semispinalis cervicis muscle activity in patients with chronic nonspecific neck pain and pain-free controls. Given that the synaptic input is distributed partly independently to different fascicles of the semispinalis cervicis muscle[21] and that changes in the structure and function of the deep spinal muscles can occur uniquely at painful segments of the spine,[22,23] it was hypothesized that changes in activation of the semispinalis cervicis may differ between spinal levels. Therefore, the aim of this study was to measure electromyograph (EMG) activity of the semispinalis cervicis during a multidirectional isometric task and PPDT at 2 spinal levels (C2 and C5). The knowledge obtained from this study may further our understanding of changes in the behavior of the deep cervical muscles in people with neck pain and the variability of change in muscle activation observed across patients.

MATERIALS AND METHODS

Patients

Ten women (age, mean ± SD: 34.1 ± 8.8 y; height: 168.4 ± 7.4 cm; weight: 68.0 ± 23.1 kg) with chronic nonspecific neck pain participated in this study. The cause of neck pain varied and included motor vehicle accident (4), work accident (2), fall (3), and a hit with a club (1).

Patients were included if they were aged between 18 and 45 years with a history of neck pain for > 6 months (mean ± SD: 9.9 ± 11.0 y), and pain intensity (average over the last week) > 2 on a 10 cm visual analogue scale. The patients' average score for the Neck Disability Index (0 to 50) (Vernon and Mior,[24]) was (mean ± SD) 19.6 ± 7.5 (range: 10 to 31) and their pain intensity was (mean ± SD) 6.1 ± 2.0 (range: 2.8 to 8.0).

Nine pain-free women (age, mean ± SD: 27.2 ± 4.1 y; height: 167.2 ± 7.8 0 cm; weight: 58.6 ± 7.1 kg) were recruited as controls. The 2 groups did not differ in age, weight, or height (P > 0.05). Controls subjects were included if they had no relevant history of neck pain or injury that limited their function and/or required treatment from a health professional. Participants were excluded from both groups if they had any major circulatory, neurological, respiratory disorders, recent or current pregnancies, or previous spinal surgery. The sample size was limited to 10 patients per group because of the invasive nature of the EMG procedure that is in line with previous studies using similar techniques.[25,26] Data from one of the 10 control was discarded because of low signal quality. Ethical approval for the study was granted by the Regional Ethics Committee (reference number-20090039). Informed written consent of the procedures was collected from all patients in accordance to the Declaration of Helsinki.

PPDT

PPDT was measured with an electronic algometer (Somedic Production, Stockholm, Sweden) over the C2-C3 and C5-C6 zygapophyseal joints. Patients were measured on their most painful side (right side for 8 patients) and healthy controls were measured on the right side. The algometer probe tip (1 cm²) was applied to the skin at a rate of 30 kPa/s and the participant was instructed to depress a handheld switch at their first perception of pain, at which point the application of pressure ceased. PPDT measures have demonstrated reliability[27] and validity[28] at different regions of the spine.[29,30] An explanation of the PPDT measurement procedure, followed by a demonstration on the forearm or thigh of the participant was performed before 4 consecutive PPDT measures at each location. The first PPDT measure was discarded because it is reported to be higher than the subsequent measures, and the mean of the subsequent 3 PPDT measures was used for further analysis.[31]

EMG

Intramuscular EMG was recorded from the semispinalis cervicis muscle unilaterally at the levels of the second (C2) and fifth spinous process (C5) on the same side where PPDT was assessed. Patients were measured on the side of greatest pain as atrophy of the deep lumbar multifidus muscle was shown predominantly ipsilateral to the symptoms in patients with low-back pain.[22,23] Furthermore, some studies have shown greater muscle dysfunction ipsilateral to the side of pain in patients with unilateral CNP compared with the nonpainful side.[32] Healthy controls were measured on the right side.

Wire electrodes made of teflon-coated stainless steel (diameter: 0.1 mm; A-M Systems, Carlsborg, WA) were inserted in the semispinalis cervicis by a 27-G hypodermic needle. Approximately 3 to 4 mm of insulation was removed from the tip of the wires to obtain an interference EMG signal.

Needle insertion was guided by ultrasound using a 10 MHz linear transducer (Acuson 128 Computed Sonography, Canada).[25] Ultrasound is a reliable tool to visualize the deep cervical extensors as shown by measurements of cross-sectional area.[34,35] Participants were lying prone on a treatment table with the head resting in a neutral position. The spinous process of C2 was located by palpation as the first bony landmark caudal to the occiput.[35] The spinous process of C5 was identified by palpation counting from C2 downwards and checked by counting upwards from C7 that was palpated as the most prominent spinous process.[36]

Cutaneous landmarks were marked with a pen to locate a point 1.5 cm lateral to the median line of the second and fifth cervical spinous process as the insertion point for the semispinalis cervicis.[37] The ultrasound transducer was placed transversally in the midline over C2 and C5, and moved laterally to image the extensor muscles. The identification of the echogenic (bright, reflective) laminae and the spinous process are the main bony landmarks used to identify the cervical extensors that are separated by echogenic fascia layers.[33,38]

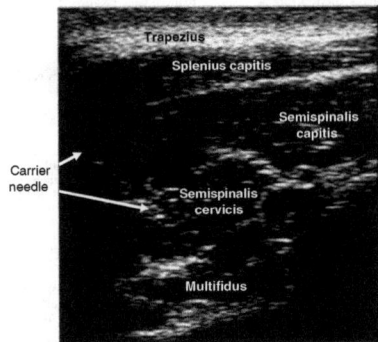

FIGURE 1. Ultrasound image of the neck extensors (right side) with the carrier needle inserted into the semispinalis cervicis at the level of C5.

Needle insertion started after clear identification of semispinalis cervicis muscle and after disinfection of the skin (injection swabs: 70% isopropylalkohol, 30 × 30 mm, Selefatrade, Spånga, Sweden). Then the needle containing the wire was inserted vertically into the muscle belly,[37] the right location checked by ultrasonography (Fig. 1), and the needle removed immediately leaving the wire in the muscle for the duration of the experiment.

Intramuscular EMG activity was acquired in monopolar mode. Two common reference electrodes were placed around the right and left wrist. EMG signals were amplified (EMG-USB2, 256-channel EMG amplifier, OT Bioelettronica, Torino, Italy; 500 to 5 kHz), sampled at 10,000 Hz, and converted to digital form by a 12-bit analog-to-digital converter.

Procedure

Participants were first positioned in prone for PPDT measurement, followed by insertion of the wire electrodes into the semispinalis cervicis. Participants were then seated in a device for the measurement of multidirectional neck force (Aalborg University, Denmark)[14] with their head secured in a padded head-brace. The back was supported; the torso was securely strapped to the backrest, the knees and hips were positioned with 90 degrees of flexion, and the hands rested on the thighs. The multidirectional neck force–

recording apparatus is equipped with 8 adjustable contacts that are fastened around the head to provide resistance during cervical isometric contractions. The adjustable contacts are equipped with transducers (strain gauges) to allow force measures in the sagittal and coronal planes. The electrical signals from the strain gauges were amplified (OT Bioelettronica) and their output displayed on an oscilloscope as visual feedback to the patient.

After a period of familiarization with the measuring device and a period to practice the desired contractions, participants performed contractions in the horizontal plane, first at 15-N and then at 30-N force with change in force direction in the range 0 to 360 degrees (circular contractions; 0 degrees: flexion, 90 degrees: right lateral flexion, 180 degrees: extension, 270 degrees: left lateral flexion). Real-time visual feedback of force direction and magnitude was provided on an oscilloscope positioned in front of the patient. A 15- or 30-N circle template was superimposed on the oscilloscope to guide the participants through the circular contractions. Participants were able to practice the circular motion with no load. After a 5-minute rest period, the patients performed the 15-N followed by the 30-N contractions. Each circular contraction consisted of 1 clockwise and 1 counterclockwise contraction. The contractions were performed as a continuous motion over a 12-second interval, as guided by a counter. Each circular contraction was separated by rest periods of 2 minutes.

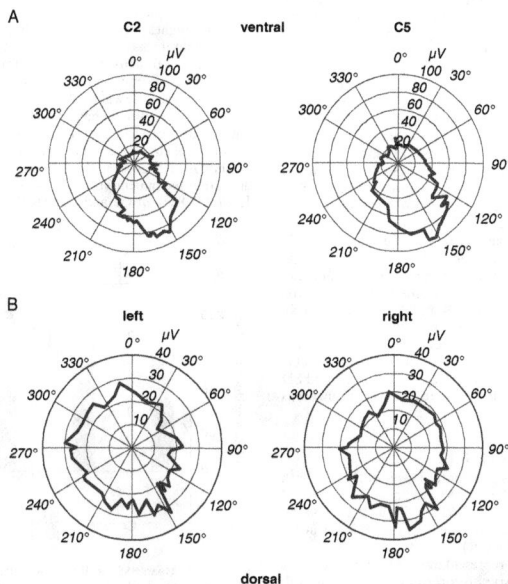

FIGURE 2. Representative directional activation curves of the semispinalis cervicis muscle at the spinal levels C2 and C5 for a 15-N contraction during a clockwise circular contraction for (A) a healthy control and (B) a patient with neck pain.

Signal Analysis

The amplitude of the EMG was estimated as the average rectified value (ARV) of the signal in non-overlapping intervals of 250 ms. The ARV of the EMG as a function of the angle of force direction will be referred to in the following as directional activation curves.[14] The directional activation curves represent the modulation in intensity of muscle activity with the direction of force exertion and represent a closed area when expressed in polar coordinates. A line connecting the origin with the central point of this area is defined as a directional vector, with the vector length expressed as a percentage of the mean ARV of the EMG during the entire circular contraction. This normalized vector length represents the specificity of muscle activation: it is equal to 0 if the muscle is active in the same way in all directions and, conversely, it corresponds to 100% if the muscle is active in exclusively 1 direction. In addition, the ARV EMG was averaged across the entire circular contraction to provide an estimate of total muscle activity. No differences in EMG were found for the clockwise and counterclockwise task, so the data were combined to obtain an average EMG ARV. One EMG recording from the semispinalis cervicis at the level of C5 in a healthy control was lost because of inadequate signal quality and therefore, the EMG data from C5 was excluded for this participant.

Statistical Analysis

Before statistical comparison, all data were tested for normal distribution by the Kolmogorov-Smirnov test and normality was confirmed. A 2-way analysis of variance (ANOVA) was used to assess differences in PPDT, with location (C2, C5) as the within-subject variable and group (patient, control) as the between-subject variable. Furthermore, 3-way ANOVAs were used to assess differences in the directional specificity of semispinalis cervicis activity (vector length) and the average ARV obtained across the entire circular contraction, with force (15, 30 N) and location (C2, C5) as the within-subject variables and group (patient, control) as the between-subject variable. Significant differences revealed by ANOVA were followed by post hoc Student-Newman-Keuls pair-wise comparisons.

Linear regression analysis was conducted on PPDT, and (1) directional specificity of semispinalis cervicis activity (average of 15- and 30-N contractions); and (2) mean activity of the semispinalis cervicis muscle during the circular contractions (average of 15- and 30-N contractions). Furthermore, regression analysis was conducted between the directional specificity and mean EMG activity of the semispinalis cervicis muscle (data pooled across all patients and healthy controls). Results are reported as mean and SD in the text and SE in the figures. Statistical significance was set at $P < 0.05$.

RESULTS

Patients displayed significantly lower PPDTs at both levels (C2: 71.4 ± 34.5 kPa; C5: 83.1 ± 38.7 kPa) compared with controls (C2: 128.0 ± 43.4 kPa; C5: 169.9 ± 57.4 kPa; $P < 0.01$). Across both groups the PPDT were lower at C2 compared with C5 ($P < 0.001$).

Figure 2 illustrates representative semispinalis cervicis directional activation curves recorded at the levels of both C2 and C5 during a circular contraction performed at 15 N for a representative healthy control and a patient. In this example, the healthy control presents with defined

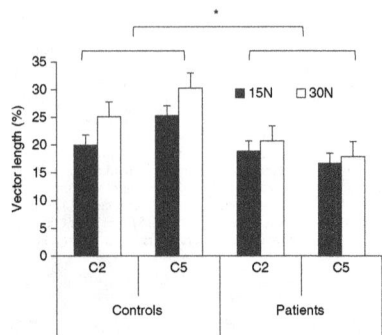

FIGURE 3. Mean ± SE of the directional specificity (vector length) of the semispinalis cervicis muscle for pain-free controls and patients with neck pain performing a circular contraction in the horizontal plane at 15 and 30 N with change in force direction in the range 0 to 360 degrees. The vector length is expressed as a percentage of the mean average rectified value during the entire task: 100% means that the electromyograph amplitude is different from 0 in exclusively 1 direction (ideal specificity).

activation of the semispinalis cervicis at both spinal levels with the highest amplitude of activity towards extension with a slight ipsilateral posterolateral direction. Conversely, the directional activation curves for the representative patient indicate more even-activation levels of the semispinalis cervicis muscle in all directions.

Values of directional specificity in the EMG of the semispinalis cervicis muscle did not differ between the 15- or 30-N circular contractions or spinal level. However, as shown in Figure 3, the directional specificity was less defined in the patient group for both the 15 N (mean ± SD: $18.87 \pm 7.88\%$ at C2 and $16.69 \pm 7.24\%$ at C5) and 30-N

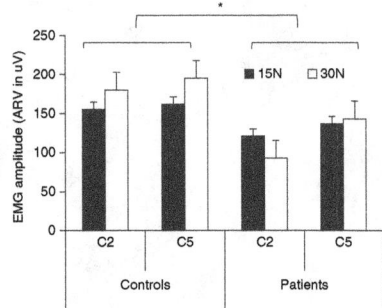

FIGURE 4. Mean ± SE of the mean electromyograph activity [average rectified value (ARV)] of the semispinalis cervicis muscle for healthy controls and patients with neck pain performing a circular contraction in the horizontal plane at 15 and 30 N with change in force direction in the range 0 to 360 degrees.

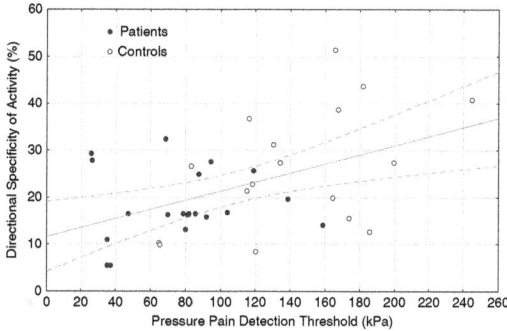

FIGURE 5. Scatter plot showing the correlation between the pressure pain detection threshold and directional specificity of semispinalis cervicis activity ($R^2 = 0.22$, $P < 0.05$). Dashed lines represent the 95% confidence interval.

circular contractions ($20.74 \pm 7.22\%$ at C2 and $17.91 \pm 9.25\%$ at C5) compared with pain-free controls ($19.96 \pm 14.06\%$ at C2 and $25.20 \pm 13.85\%$ at C5 for 15 N and $25.13 \pm 14.53\%$ and $30.33 \pm 14.72\%$ at C2 and C5, respectively, for 30 N) ($F = 6.17$; $P < 0.05$).

Likewise, the patients demonstrated lower values of ARV (averaged across the circular contractions) for the semispinalis cervicis during the circular contractions performed at both 15 N ($121.07 \pm 62.07\,\mu V$ at C2 and $136.95 \pm 53.09\,\mu V$ at C5) and 30 N ($110.61 \pm 39.02\,\mu V$ at C2 and $143.04 \pm 63.57\,\mu V$ at C5) compared with controls ($155.34 \pm 70.28\,\mu V$ at C2 and $162.03 \pm 52.01\,\mu V$ at C5 for 15 N and $180.05 \pm 85.48\,\mu V$ at C2 and $195.22 \pm 64.31\,\mu V$ at C5 for 30 N) ($F = 9.7$; $P < 0.01$, Fig. 4). The ARV of the semispinalis cervicis did not differ between the 15- and 30-N circular contractions at both spinal levels (both $P > 0.05$).

When the patient and control data were pooled together, a significant relation was identified between the PPDT and directional specificity of semispinalis cervicis

activity ($R^2 = 0.22$, $P < 0.05$; Fig. 5), and between PPDT and mean activity ($R^2 = 0.15$, $P < 0.05$; Fig. 6). The mean activity of the semispinalis cervicis and directional specificity were also significantly correlated ($R^2 = 0.41$, $P < 0.05$; Fig. 7). Table 1 presents the results of the linear regression analysis for all comparisons for both the patient and the control group.

DISCUSSION

As expected, the PPDT over the C2 and C5 zygapophyseal joints was significantly lower in women with CNP compared with controls. This study also found lower EMG amplitude and lower directional specificity of the semispinalis cervicis at these spinal levels during multidirectional isometric contractions of the neck. Moreover, evidence of a correlation between PPDT and EMG activity, and PPDT and directional specificity of the semispinalis cervicis was found.

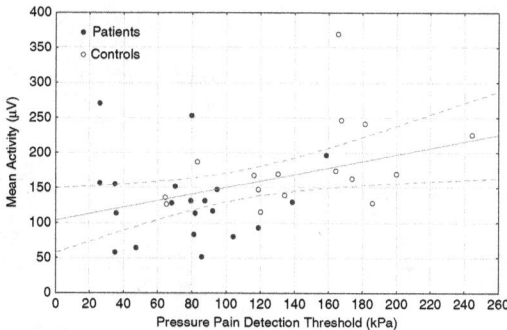

FIGURE 6. Scatter plot showing the correlation between pressure pain detection threshold and semispinalis cervicis mean electromyograph amplitude ($R^2 = 0.15$, $P < 0.05$). Dashed lines represent the 95% confidence interval.

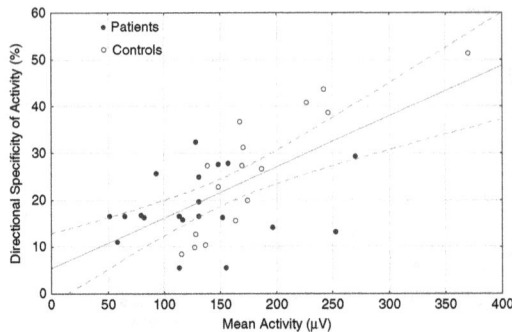

FIGURE 7. Scatter plot showing the correlation between semispinalis cervicis mean electromyograph amplitude and directional specificity ($R^2 = 0.41$, $P < 0.05$). Dashed lines represent the 95% confidence interval.

EMG Amplitude and Directional Specificity

Consistent with previous findings,[8] this study showed reduced and less-defined activity of the semispinalis cervicis muscle in patients with neck pain compared with pain-free controls. Previously, the activity of the semispinalis cervicis was investigated at the level of C3,[8] whereas in this study we further investigated the activation of the semispinalis cervicis at the levels C2 and C5. Lower activity of the semispinalis cervicis (and multifidus), as measured with muscle functional magnetic resonance imaging, was also found in patients with mechanical neck pain when assessed at the levels C5-C6 and C7-T1 during cervical extension with the head positioned in a neutral position.[9] The observation that the semispinalis cervicis muscle was similarly altered across different spinal levels, suggests a generalized change in activation in all fascicles rather than a change localized to a specific segment. Localized changes in muscle structure has been shown to occur specifically at painful segments of the spine,[22,23] although generalized changes in muscle composition that are not isolated to 1 level of the spine have been demonstrated. For example, in patients with persistent whiplash-induced neck pain, fatty infiltration of the neck extensors was observed across several spinal levels (C3-C7).[39] In addition, relatively smaller cross-sectional area of the semispinalis cervicis was also noted across all levels.[40] In the present study, the most painful segment was not specifically investigated; therefore, further investigations are required to reveal the extent or distribution patterns of altered EMG activity across spinal levels with respect to the painful segments.

The less-defined activation of the semispinalis cervicis muscle in patients with neck pain during the multidirectional isometric task is in accordance with decreased directional specificity found for the sternocleidomastoid,[14] and splenius capitis[5] muscles in patients with neck pain. Lower specificity of neck muscle activity may be interpreted as a functional adaptation or possibly maladaptation to pain and might reflect impaired neural drive to the neck muscles in patients.[14] It may represent an attempt to increase cervical spine stability similar to coactivation of cervical muscles[41–43] by activating muscles over a larger range of motion. This multidirectional activation of the cervical muscles could provide muscle tension when moving in all directions which would support cervical stability, even though the overall EMG amplitude of semispinalis cervicis was reduced in patients compared with pain-free controls.

PPDT

The findings of lower PPDT over the zygapophyseal joints C2 and C5 in patients as compared with asymptomatic individuals, is consistent with previous investigations over cervical joints[44] and muscles.[45] The increased sensitivity to pressure, as was found at C2 and C5, is likely to explain the frequent reports of pain at these locations.[46] For example, in a study of patients after a whiplash injury, half who reported headache localized the source of their

TABLE 1. Results of the Linear Regression Analysis (R^2) Between Pressure Pain Detection Threshold (PPDT) and Directional Specificity and Mean EMG Activity for Both the Patient and the Control Group Separated and Taken Together

	Patients		Controls		Patients + Controls	
	Dir. Spec.	Mean Activity	Dir. Spec.	Mean Activity	Dir. Spec.	Mean Activity
PPDT at C2	0.12	0.13	0.16	0.13	0.06	0.04
PPDT at C5	0.26	0.04	0.20	0.24	*0.28*	*0.46*
PPDT at C2 + C5	0.01	0.01	0.22	0.17	*0.22*	*0.15*

Bold and italic indicates significant correlation: $P < 0.05$.
Dir. Spec. indcates direction specificity; PPDT, pressure pain detection threshold.

     © 2013 Lippincott Williams & Wilkins

pain to the C2-C3 zygapophyseal joint area.[47] In addition, mechanical palpation over the zygapophyseal joints from C0 to C4, but not C5-C7, was significantly more painful in patients with headache symptoms compared with pain-free controls.[48] Lower PPDT may occur as a result of local changes in the periphery such as higher serotonin (5-HT) and glutamate found in the interstitial fluid of upper trapezius muscle of patients with work-related trapezius myalgia.[49] Central sensitization, however, contributes significantly[44,50] and generally leads to hypersensitivity to pressure.[51–53] Other components of pain, such as psychological distress (cognitive evaluative), however, do not appear to be correlated to pressure sensitivity (PPDT) in the neck of patients with nontraumatic neck-shoulder pain.[54]

As a general finding, the PPDT over the zygapophyseal joint at C2 was lower than at C5 in both groups. This suggests that C2 is more sensitive to mechanical stimulation or palpation than C5, and is in line with the observation of increasing PPDT values from C6 to T4 and T6-L4 in asymptomatic volunteers.[29] The differences between levels C2 and C5, however, are small and below the SEM (20.5 kPa) and the minimum detectable change (47.2 kPa) of PPDT of the upper trapezius muscle.[55] Thus, although a statistical difference between levels was observed in this study, the clinical relevance of the difference between both levels is unknown.

The lower values of PPDT over C2 compared with C5 suggest that PPDT reflects the sensitivity and tenderness of the tissues to pressure and not the pain report by the patient.[56] Indeed, only a weak correlation has been shown between PPDT over the cervical spinous process and intensity of subacute neck pain after a whiplash injury.[57] It has been proposed[58] that C2 may be more vulnerable to loads because of the mechanical stress that results from movement coupling of the upper (C0-C3) and the lower (C2-C7) cervical spine.[59]

Relation Between PPDT and EMG Measures

In this study, a correlation between PPDT and EMG amplitude and PPDT and directional specificity of the semispinalis cervicis was found when patient and control data were pooled. To date, few studies have investigated correlations between PPDT and EMG amplitude in patients with pain or in healthy controls. In patients with masseter muscle pain, PPDT was not only lower in the masseter muscle when compared with pain-free controls, but there was also a correlation between PPDT and the duration of masseter EMG activity during biting tasks of hard foods. However, there was no correlation between PPDT of the masseter and maximum biting force.[31] The results from this study imply that during functional tasks, PPDT may have a greater influence on muscle activity patterns.

In this study, PPDT was only weakly correlated to EMG amplitude and directional specificity of the semispinalis cervicis muscle. This is supported by the observation that the correlation was not evident when analyzing each group alone. This suggests that other factors are contributing to the variability of activation of the semispinalis cervicis during the multidirectional isometric task. For example, general psychological distress and fear avoidance behavior have a strong influence on motor control.[60] Other factors such as disuse may also contribute to altered muscle activation.

Methodological Considerations

The invasive procedure of electrode placement restricted the sample size in this study as in other studies with similar procedures.[25] The small number of patients and the interindividual variability of the data resulted in nonsignificant correlations when the data were analyzed within each group making it necessary to pool the data of both groups to increase the sample size. Although no significant difference in age or weight were observed between the groups, there was a tendency for greater weight and older age in the patient group that may need to be taken into consideration. Furthermore, the EMG amplitude, directional specificity, and PPDT might have been influenced by personal factors such as activity level, comorbidity, and medication that were not monitored in this study.

Clinical Implications

The deep cervical flexors and extensors form a muscular sleeve enclosing and supporting the cervical spine.[61] Lower activation of the deep muscles during movements of the head might compromise cervical spine stability and increase the risk of injury and pain.[7,62,63] As such, specific exercises aimed at activating these deep muscles are considered essential, especially in the early phase of rehabilitation[64] in patients with either acute or chronic neck pain when high-load exercises may increase pain.[65,66] Such low-load exercises have shown efficacy for reducing pain and perceived disability.[18,67–70] Studies on the efficacy of low-load exercises for the cervical extensor muscles, however, are lacking and it remains to be determined whether motor rehabilitation exercises can reestablish directional specificity of muscle activity in patients with neck pain, and whether this would be associated with an improved outcome.

CONCLUSIONS

PPDT over the zygapophyseal joints C2 and C5 and EMG amplitude, and directional specificity of the semispinalis cervicis at the same spinal levels were significantly lower in patients with CNP compared with healthy controls. PPDT of patients and controls together correlated weakly, but significantly, with EMG mean activity and directional specificity of semispinalis cervicis suggesting that changes in the behavior of this muscle are partially related to pressure pain sensitivity. Further research is needed to fully ascertain the clinical relevance of these results and to determine whether retraining semispinalis cervicis muscle activity and directional specificity will reduce neck pain and improve patient outcome.

REFERENCES

1. Sterling M, Jull G, Vicenzino B, et al. Development of motor system dysfunction following whiplash injury. *Pain.* 2003;103:65–73.
2. Johnston V, Jull G, Souvlis T, et al. Neck movement and muscle activity characteristics in female office workers with neck pain. *Spine.* 2008;33:555–563.
3. Kumar S, Narayan Y, Prasad N, et al. Cervical electromyogram profile differences between patients of neck pain and control. *Spine.* 2007;32:E246–E253.
4. Szeto GPY, Straker LM, O'Sullivan PB. A comparison of symptomatic and asymptomatic office workers performing monotonous keyboard work—1: neck and shoulder muscle recruitment patterns. *Man Ther.* 2005;10:270–280.

5. Lindstrøm R, Schomacher J, Farina D, et al. Association between neck muscle coactivation, pain, and strength in women with neck pain. *Man Ther*. 2011;16:80–86.
6. Edmonston SJ, Björnsdóttir G, Pálsson T, et al. Endurance and fatigue characteristics of the neck flexor and extensor muscles during isometric tests in patients with postural neck pain. *Man Ther*. 2011;16:332–338.
7. Falla D, Jull G, Hodges PW. Patients with neck pain demonstrate reduced electromyographic activity of the deep cervical flexor muscles during performance of the craniocervical flexion test. *Spine*. 2004;29:2108–2114.
8. Schomacher J, Farina D, Lindstroem R, et al. Chronic trauma-induced neck pain impairs the neural control of the deep semispinalis cervicis muscle. *Clin Neurophysiol*. 2012;123:1403–1408.
9. O'Leary S, Cagnie B, Reeve A, et al. Is there altered activity of the extensor muscles in chronic mechanical neck pain? A functional magnetic resonance imaging study. *Arch Phys Med Rehabil*. 2011;92:929–934.
10. Falla D, O'Leary S, Farina D, et al. Association between intensity of pain and impairment in onset and activation of the deep cervical flexors in patients with persistent neck pain. *Clin J Pain*. 2011;27:309–314.
11. Lund JP, Donga R, Widmer CG, et al. The pain-adaptation model: a discussion of the relationship between musculoskeletal pain and motor activity. *Can J Physiol Pharmacol*. 1991;49:683–694.
12. Graven-Nielsen T, Svensson P, Arendt-Nielsen L. Effects of experimental muscle pain on muscle activity and co-ordination during static and dynamic motor function. *Electroencephalogr Clin Neurophysiol*. 1997;10:156–164.
13. Birch L, Christensen H, Arendt-Nielsen L, et al. The influence of experimental muscle pain on motor unit activity during low-level contraction. *Eur J Appl Physiol*. 2000;83:200–206.
14. Falla D, Lindstrøm R, Rechter L, et al. Effect of pain on modulation in discharge rate of sternocleidomastoid motor units with force direction. *Clin Neurophysiol*. 2010;121:744–753.
15. Nijs J, Daenen L, Cras P, et al. Nociception affects motor output: a review on sensory-motor interaction with focus on clinical implications. *Clin J Pain*. 2012;28:175–181.
16. Hodges PW, Tucker K. Moving differently in pain: a new theory to explain the adaptation to pain. *Pain*. 2011;152:S90–S98.
17. Ylinen J, Nykänen M, Kautiainen H, et al. Evaluation of repeatability of pressure algometry on the neck muscles for clinical use. *Man Ther*. 2007;12:192–197.
18. O'Leary S, Falla D, Hodges PW, et al. Specific therapeutic exercise of the neck induces immediate local hypoalgesia. *J Pain*. 2007;8:832–839.
19. Walton D, MacDermid J, Nielson W, et al. Pressure pain threshold testing demonstrates predictive ability in people with acute whiplash. *J Orthop Sport Phys Ther*. 2011;41:658–665.
20. Walton D, MacDermid J, Nielson W, et al. A descriptive study of pressure pain threshold at 2 standardized sites in people with acute or subacute neck pain. *J Orthop Sport Phys Ther*. 2011;41:651–657.
21. Schomacher J, Dideriksen JL, Farina D, et al. Recruitment of motor units in two fascicles of the semispinalis cervicis muscle. *J Neurophysiol*. 2012;107:3078–3085.
22. Wallwork TL, Stanton WR, Freke M, et al. The effect of chronic low back pain on size and contraction of the lumbar multifidus muscle. *Man Ther*. 2009;14:496–500.
23. Hides J, Gilmore C, Stanton W, et al. Multifidus size and symmetry among chronic LBP and healthy asymptomatic subjects. *Man Ther*. 2008;13:43–49.
24. Vernon H, Mior S. The neck disability index: a study of reliability and validity. *J Manipulative and Physiological Therapeutics*. 1991;14:409–415.
25. Bexander CSM, Mellor R, Hodges PW. Effect of gaze direction on neck muscle activity during cervical rotation. *Exp Brain Res*. 2005;167:422–432.
26. Blouin J-S, Siegmund GP, Carpenter MG, et al. Neural control of superficial and deep neck muscles in humans. *J Neurophysiol*. 2007;98:920–928.
27. Nussbaum EL, Daownes L. Reliability of clinical pressure-pain algometric measurments obtained on consecutive days. *Phys Ther*. 1998;78:160–169.
28. Kinser AM, Sands WA, Stone MH. Reliability and validity of a pressure algometer. *J Strength Cond Res*. 2009;23:312–314.
29. Keating L, Lubke C, Powell V, et al. Mid-thoracic tenderness: a comparison of pressure pain threshold between spinal regions, in asymptomatic subjects. *Man Ther*. 2001;6:34–39.
30. Schenk P, Laeubli T, Klipstein A. Validity of pressure pain thresholds in female workers with and without recurrent low back pain. *Eur Spine J*. 2007;16:267–275.
31. Shiau YY, Peng CC, Wen SC, et al. The effects of masseter muscle pain on biting performance. *J Oral Rehabil*. 2003;30:978–984.
32. Falla D, Jull G, Rainoldi A, et al. Neck flexor muscle fatigue is side specific in patients with unilateral neck pain. *Eur J Pain*. 2004;8:71–77.
33. Stokes M, Hides J, Elliott JM, et al. Rehabilitative ultrasound imaging of the posterior paraspinal muscles. *J Orthop Sport Phys Ther*. 2007;37:581–595.
34. Kristjansson E. Reliability of ultrasonography for the cervical multifidus muscle in asymptomatic and symptomatic subjects. *Man Ther*. 2004;9:83–88.
35. Lee JP, Tseng WY, Shau YW, et al. Measurement of segmental cervical multifidus contraction by ultrasonography in asymptomatic adults. *Man Ther*. 2007;12:286–294.
36. Robinson R, Robinson HS, Bjørke G, et al. Reliability and validity of a palpation tecnique for identifying the spinous processes of C7 and L5. *Man Ther*. 2009;14:409–414.
37. Kramer M, Schmid I, Sander S, et al. Guidelines for the intramuscular positioning of EMG electrodes in the semispinalis capitis and cervicis muscles. *J Electromyogr Kinesiol*. 2003;13:289–295.
38. Whittaker JL, Teyhen DS, Elliott JM, et al. Rehabilitative ultrasound imaging: understanding the technology and its applications. *J Orthop Sport Phys Ther*. 2007;37:434–449.
39. Elliott JM, Jull G, Noteboom JT, et al. Fatty infiltration in the cervical extensor muscles in persistent whiplash-associated disorders: a magnetic resonance imaging analysis. *Spine*. 2006;31:E847–E855.
40. Elliott JM, Jull G, Noteboom JT, et al. MRI study of the cross-sectional area for the cervical extensor musculature in patients with persistent whiplash associated disorders (WAD). *Man Ther*. 2008;13:258–265.
41. Lee PJ, Rogers EL, Granata KP. Active trunk stiffness increases with co-contraction. *J Electromyogr Kinesiol*. 2006;16:51–57.
42. Cheng C-H, Lin K-H, Wang J-L. Co-contraction of cervical muscles during sagittal and coronal neck motions at different movement speeds. *Eur J Appl Physiol*. 2008;103:647–654.
43. Fernández-de-las-Peñas C, Falla D, Arendt-Nielsen L, et al. Cervical muscle co-activation in isometric contractions is enhanced in chronic tension-type headache patients. *Cephalalgia*. 2008;28:744–751.
44. Javanshir K, Ortega-Santiago R, Mohseni-Bandpei MA, et al. Exploration of somatosensory impairments in subjects with mechanical idiopathick neck pain: a preliminary study. *J Manipulative Physiol Ther*. 2010;33:493–499.
45. Kasch H, Stengaard-Pedersen K, Arendt-Nielsen L, et al. Pain thresholds and tenderness in neck and head following acute whiplash injury: a prospective study. *Cephalalgia*. 2001;21:189–197.
46. Bogduk N, McGuirk B. *Management of Acute and Chronic Neck Pain, An Evidence-based Approach*. Edinburgh: Elsevier; 2006.
47. Lord S, Barnsley L, Wallis BJ, et al. Chronic cervical zygapophysial joint pain after whiplash. *Spine*. 1996;21:1737–1745.
48. Jull G, Amiri M, Bullock-Saxton J, et al. Cervical musculoskeletal impairment in frequent intermittent headache. Part 1:

Subjects with single headaches. *Cephalalgia.* 2007;27: 793–802.
49. Rosendahl L, Larsson B, Kristiansen J, et al. Increase in muscle nociceptive substances and anaerobic metabolism in patients with trapezius myalgia: microdialysis in rest and during exercise. *Pain.* 2004;112:324–334.
50. Gerdle B, Lemming D, Kristiansen J, et al. Biochemical alterations in the trapezius muscle of patients with chronic whiplash associated disorders (WAD)—a microdialysis study. *Eur J Pain.* 2008;12:82–93.
51. Schmid A, Brunner F, Wright A, et al. Paradigm shift in manual therapy? Evidence for a central nervous system component in the response to passive cervical joint mobilisation. *Man Ther.* 2008;13:387–396.
52. Nijs J, Van Houdenhove B. From acute musculoskeletal pain to chronic widespread pain and fibromyalgia: application of pain neurophysiology in manual therapy practice. *Man Ther.* 2009;14:3–12.
53. Nijs J, Van Houdenhove B, Oostendorp RAB. Recognition of central sensitization in patients with musculoskeletal pain: application of pain neurophysiology in manual therapy practice. *Man Ther.* 2010;15:135–141.
54. Sjörs A, Larsson B, Persson A, et al. An increased response to experimental muscle pain is related to psychological status in women with chronic non-traumatic neck-shoulder pain. *BMC Musculoskelet Disord.* 2011;12:230.
55. Walton D, MacDermid J, Nielson W, et al. Reliability, standard error, and minimum detectable change of clinical pressure pain threshold testing in people with and without acute neck pain. *J Orthop Sport Phys Ther.* 2011;41: 644–650.
56. Jensen K, Andersen HØ, Olesen J, et al. Pressure-pain threshold in human temporal region. Evaluation of a new pressure algometer. *Pain.* 1986;25:313–323.
57. Kamper SJ, Maher CG, Hush JM, et al. Relationship between pressure pain thresholds and pain ratings in patients with whiplash-associated disorders. *Clin J Pain.* 2011;27:495–501.
58. Wolf HD. Bewegungssegment C2/3—auch eine Übergangsregion der Wirbelsäule [Movement segment C2-C3—also a

transitional zone of the spine]. *Manuelle Medizin.* 1997;35: 59–62.
59. White AA, Panjabi MM. Clinical Biomechanics of the Spine. Philadelphia: J. B. Lippincott Company; 1990.
60. Oddsdottir GL, Kristjansson E. Two different courses of impaired cervical kinaesthesia following a whiplash injury. A one-year prospective study. *Man Ther.* 2012;17:60–65.
61. Mayoux-Benhamou MA, Revel M, Vallee C. Selective electromyography of dorsal neck muscles in humans. *Exp Brain Res.* 1997;113:353–360.
62. Cholewicki J, McGill SM. Mechanical stability of the *in vivo* lumbar spine: implications for injury and chronic low back pain. *Clin Biomech.* 1996;11:1–15.
63. Pearson AM, Ivanicic PC, Ito S, et al. Facet joint kinematics and injury mechanisms during simulated whiplash. *Spine.* 2004;29:390–397.
64. O'Leary S, Falla D, Elliott JM, et al. Muscle dysfunction in cervical spine pain: implications for assessment and management. *J Orthop Sport Phys Ther.* 2009;39:324–333.
65. Jull G, Sterling M, Falla D, et al. *Whiplash, Headache, and Neck Pain: Research-Based Directions for Physical Therapies.* Edinburgh: Churchill Livingstone (Elsevier); 2008.
66. Jull G. Übungsansatz bei HWS-Störungen: Wie fließen die Ergebnisse der Forschung in die Praxis ein? [An exercise approach for cervical disorders: How does research inform practice?] *Manuelle Therapie.* 2009;13:110–116.
67. Jull G, Trott P, Potter H, et al. A randomized controlled trial of exercise and manipulative therapy for cervicogenic headache. *Spine.* 2002;27:1835–1843.
68. O'Leary S, Falla D, Jull G, et al. Muscle specificity in tests of cervical flexor muscle performance. *J Electromyogr Kinesiol.* 2007;17:35–40.
69. Jull G, Falla D, Treleaven J, et al. A therapeutic exercise approach for cervical disorders. In: Boyling JD, Jull G, eds. *Grieve's Modern Manual Therapy: The Vertebral Column.* 3rd ed. Edinburgh: Elsevier; 2004:451–470.
70. Sterling M, Jull G, Wright A. Cervical mobilisation: concurrent effects on pain, sympathetic nervous system activity and motor activity. *Man Ther.* 2001;6:72–81.

Manual Therapy 17 (2012) 544–548

Contents lists available at SciVerse ScienceDirect

Manual Therapy

journal homepage: www.elsevier.com/math

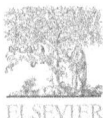

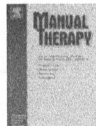

Original article

Localised resistance selectively activates the semispinalis cervicis muscle in patients with neck pain

Jochen Schomacher [a], Frank Petzke [b], Deborah Falla [b,c,*]

[a] Center for Sensory–Motor Interaction (SMI), Department of Health Science and Technology, Aalborg University, Denmark
[b] Pain Clinic, Center for Anesthesiology, Emergency and Intensive Care Medicine, University Hospital Göttingen, Göttingen, Germany
[c] Department of Neurorehabilitation Engineering, Bernstein Focus Neurotechnology Göttingen, Bernstein Center for Computational Neuroscience, University Medical Center Göttingen, Georg-August University, Göttingen, Germany

ARTICLE INFO

Article history:
Received 10 February 2012
Received in revised form
16 May 2012
Accepted 23 May 2012

Keywords:
Exercise
Semispinalis cervicis
Neck pain
EMG

ABSTRACT

The semispinalis cervicis muscle displays reduced and less defined activation in patients with neck pain which is associated with increased activity of the splenius capitis muscle. Exercises to selectively activate the semispinalis cervicis muscle may be relevant for patients with neck pain however the most appropriate type of exercise has not been determined. The purpose of this study was to investigate whether a specific exercise could selectively activate the semispinalis cervicis muscle relative to the splenius capitis. Ten women with chronic neck pain participated. Intramuscular electrodes were inserted into the semispinalis cervicis and splenius capitis unilaterally on the side of greatest pain. After testing the maximal neck extension force, three isometric exercises were performed in sitting: 1. the investigator placed a hand on the patient's occiput and pushed into flexion asking the patient to resist into extension maximally, 2. the investigator placed the thumb and index finger on the vertebral arch of C2 and pushed into flexion asking the patient to resist maximally, 3. same procedure as for C2 however the resistance was applied at C5. The ratio between the normalized electromyography (EMG) amplitude of the semispinalis cervicis and splenius capitis was computed. The relative activation of the semispinalis cervicis was greater ($P < 0.05$) than the splenius capitis with resistance at C2 (2.53 ± 2.43) compared to resistance at the occiput (1.39 ± 1.00) or at C5 (1.16 ± 0.85). The results indicate that localized resistance can achieve relative isolation of the semispinalis cervicis muscle. This exercise approach may be relevant for patients with neck pain.

© 2012 Elsevier Ltd. All rights reserved.

1. Introduction

The semispinalis cervicis is considered together with the multifidus and rotatores muscles as the deepest layer of the neck extensors (Rankin et al., 2005; Stokes et al., 2007). Together these muscles contribute towards cervical spine segmental support (Mayoux-Benhamou et al., 1997; Blouin et al., 2007) due to their relatively small moment arms (Anderson et al., 2005), attachment to adjacent vertebrae (Sommerich et al., 2000), and high proportion (~70%) of slow twitch fibres (Boyd-Clark et al., 2001).

The semispinalis cervicis muscle shows structural changes in patients with neck pain including reduced relative cross-sectional area (Elliott et al., 2008a) and fatty infiltration of muscle tissue, especially in patients with whiplash-induced neck pain (Elliott

* Corresponding author. Pain Clinic, Center for Anesthesiology, Emergency and Intensive Care Medicine, University Hospital Göttingen, Robert-Koch-Str. 40, 37075 Göttingen, Germany. Tel.: +49 (0) 551 3920109; fax: +49 (0) 551 3920110.
E-mail address: deborah.falla@bccn.uni-goettingen.de (D. Falla).

1356-689X/$ – see front matter © 2012 Elsevier Ltd. All rights reserved.
doi:10.1016/j.math.2012.05.012

et al., 2006, 2008b). In addition, a recent study has shown that the semispinalis cervicis has reduced and less defined activation during a multidirectional isometric task in patients with neck pain compared to healthy controls, i.e. it demonstrates a lower ability to produce a well-defined activation that appropriately reflects the anatomical position of the muscle relative to the spine (Schomacher et al., 2011). This electrophysiological data is supported by studies examining the deep extensors using muscle functional magnetic resonance imaging (mfMRI). The measurement of T2 shift values pre-post an isometric extension of the head in a neutral position revealed that the multifidus and semispinalis cervicis were less active in patients with mechanical neck pain compared to healthy controls (O'Leary et al., 2011). Reduced activation of the semispinalis cervicis muscle may compromise cervical spine segmental support increasing the risk of micro-/macro-trauma to the spine which may perpetuate and maintain neck pain (Pearson et al., 2004; Bogduk and McGuirk, 2006).

Reduced activation of the semispinalis cervicis in patients with neck pain together with knowledge that patients display reduced strength (Prushansky et al., 2005; Lindstrøm et al., 2011, 2012) and endurance (Lee et al., 2005) of their neck extensors supports the prescription of specific exercises to retrain the extensors in patients with neck pain (Jull et al., 2008; Elliott et al., 2010). However, the most appropriate type of exercise has not been determined (Ylinen, 2007). Since activity of the superficial extensors (e.g. splenius capitis) is frequently observed to be increased in patients with neck pain (Szeto et al., 2005; Kumar et al., 2007; Johnston et al., 2008; Lindstrøm et al., 2011), an exercise which specifically targets the semispinalis cervicis muscle is considered most appropriate (Jull et al., 2008; O'Leary et al., 2009). Thus the purpose of this study was to investigate whether specific resistance to the head or spine could selectively activate the semispinalis cervicis muscle relative to the more superficial extensor, the splenius capitis.

2. Methods

2.1. Subjects

Ten women with chronic neck pain participated in this study (Table 1). Patients were included if they were between 18 and 45 years, had a history of neck pain greater than 6 months and if their neck pain intensity (average over the last week) was greater than 2 on a 10 cm visual analogue scale (VAS). Patients were excluded if they displayed neurological signs and/or had undergone cervical spine surgery. The impact of neck pain on the patients' daily life was assessed with the Neck Disability Index (0–50) (Vernon and Mior, 1991) and their pain over the last week was assessed with a VAS. The onset of pain in eight of the patients was attributed to trauma while the other two had idiopathic pain.

Ethical approval for the study was granted by the Regional Ethics Committee (N-20090039). All participants provided written informed consent and procedures were conducted according to the Declaration of Helsinki.

2.2. Electromyography

Intramuscular electromyography (EMG) was acquired from the semispinalis cervicis and splenius capitis muscles at the level of the 3rd spinous process (C3) unilaterally on the side of greatest pain (right side for 8 patients). Wire electrodes made of Teflon-coated stainless steel (diameter: 0.1 mm; A-M Systems, Carlsborg, WA) were inserted in the muscle via a 27-gauge hypodermic needle. Approximately 3–4 mm of insulation was removed from the tip of the wires to obtain an interference EMG signal. Needle insertion was guided by ultrasound (Acuson 128 Computed Sonography, Canada) using a 10-MHz linear transducer (Bexander et al., 2005; Lee et al., 2007). Ultrasound is a reliable tool to visualize the deep neck extensors (Kristjansson, 2004; Stokes et al., 2007). Participants were positioned in prone with the head in a neutral position. The spinous

Table 1
Demographics of the 10 patients (mean ± SD).

Demographic	Mean ± SD	Range
Age (years)	31.7 ± 8.7	22–43
Height (cm)	169.4 ± 4.4	163–176
Weight (kg)	63.7 ± 15.3	48–100
VAS (0–10)	5.4 ± 1.9	2.5–8.0
NDI (0–50)	20.1 ± 6.8	9–32
Pain duration (years)	5.0 ± 2.2	1–9.0
Cause of neck pain	Trauma; $n = 8$	
	Car accident; $n = 5$	
	Bicycle accident; $n = 1$	
	Fall from a horse; $n = 1$	
	Fall; $n = 1$	
	Idiopathic; $n = 2$	

process of the second cervical vertebrae was located by palpation as the first bony landmark caudal to the occiput and a cutaneous landmark was made at the level of the third cervical spinous process (Lee et al., 2007). The ultrasound transducer was placed transversally in the midline over C3 and moved laterally to image the extensor muscles. The identification of the echogenic (bright, reflective) laminae and the spinous process are the main bony landmarks for locating the cervical extensors which are separated by echogenic fascia layers (Stokes et al., 2007). The insertion point of the needle for the semispinalis cervicis was 1.5 cm lateral to the median line and the needle was inserted vertically as previously described (Kramer et al., 2003). The insertion point for the splenius capitis was 2–3 mm caudal to the former one. The needle was inserted obliquely at a ~45° angle.

Following skin disinfection (injection swabs: 70% isopropylalkohol, 30 × 30 mm, Selefatrade, Spånga, Sweden), the needle containing the wire was inserted into the muscle belly and removed immediately leaving the wire in the muscle for the duration of the experiment. Signals were acquired in monopolar mode. Two common reference electrodes were placed around the right and left wrists. EMG signals were amplified (EMG-USB2, 256-channel EMG amplifier, OT Bioelettronica, Torino, Italy; 500 Hz–5 kHz), sampled at 10,000 Hz, and converted to digital form by a 12-bit analogue-to-digital converter.

2.3. Procedure

After electrode insertion the subject was seated with the head rigidly fixed in a device for the measurement of multidirectional neck force with the back supported, knees and hips in 90° of flexion, the torso firmly strapped to the seat back and the hands resting comfortably on the lap (Falla et al., 2010). The device is equipped with eight adjustable contacts which are fastened around the head to stabilize the head and provide resistance during isometric contractions of the neck. The force device is equipped with force transducers (strain gauges) to measure force in the sagittal and coronal planes. The electrical signals from the strain gauges were amplified (OT Bioelettronica, Torino, Italy) and their output was displayed on an oscilloscope as visual feedback to the subject. Following a period of familiarization with the measuring device, subjects performed three neck extension maximum voluntary contractions (MVC) separated by 1 min of rest. Verbal encouragement was provided to the subject. The highest value of force recorded over the 2 maximum contractions was selected as the maximal force.

Following a rest of ~10 min, the subject was seated upright comfortably on a chair with the back supported and the hands resting in a relaxed position on the thighs. The investigator was standing on the right side of the subject and fixed the ventral aspect of the subject's torso with the right hand.

Three isometric exercises were performed and each was sustained for ~5 s (Fig. 1). For the first exercise, the investigator placed his (left) hand on the occiput and pushed into flexion asking the patient to resist maximally. For the second exercise, the investigator placed the thumb and index finger of his (left) hand approximately on the vertebral arch of C2 and pushed into flexion asking the patient to resist maximally. For the third exercise the procedure was identical to that at C2 however the resistance was applied approximately at C5. Five minutes rest was provided between each exercise. Subjects had practised each contraction prior to insertion of the electrodes and then repeated each exercise twice with electrodes in situ. The peak EMG amplitude from the two contractions was taken for further analysis.

2.4. Signal analysis

The amplitude of the EMG for both the semispinalis cervicis and splenius capitis muscles was estimated as the average rectified

A   B   C

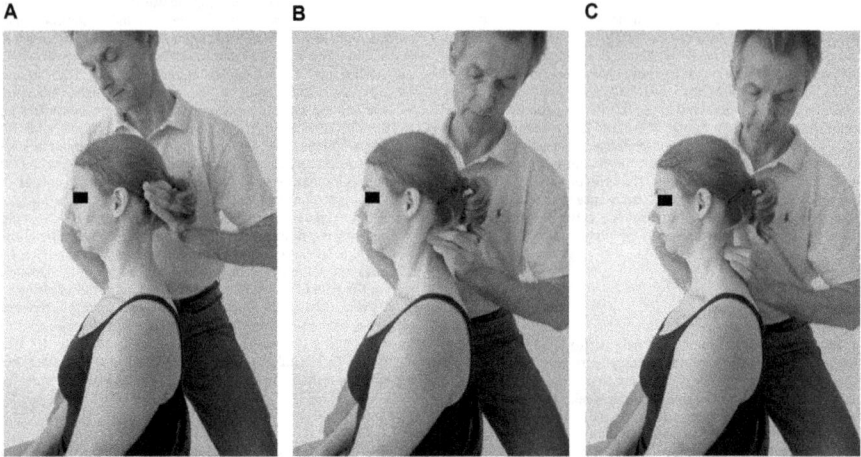

Fig. 1. Illustration of the isometric exercises with the patient pushing into extension against resistance at A) the occiput, B) C2, and C) C5. Each contraction was sustained for 5 s.

value (ARV) of the signal in non-overlapping intervals of 250 ms and averaged over the 5 s contraction. The peak ARV computed during each exercise was normalized with respect to the peak ARV obtained during the MVC and expressed as a percentage. Since the manual resistance could not be standardized across conditions, the ratio between the normalized ARV of the semispinalis cervicis and splenius capitis muscle was compared across conditions.

2.5. Statistical analysis

A one-way analysis of variance (ANOVA) was used to evaluate differences in the ratio of semispinalis cervicis and splenius capitis normalized EMG ARV between the three different conditions with location of resistance (occiput, C2 and C5) as the between subject variable. Significant differences revealed by ANOVA were followed by post-hoc Student–Newman–Keuls (SNK) pair-wise comparisons. Results are reported as mean and standard deviation (SD) in the text and standard error (SE) in the figures. Statistical significance was set at $P < 0.05$.

3. Results

The mean and SD of the ratio of semispinalis cervicis and splenius capitis normalized EMG ARV was 1.39 ± 1.00, 2.53 ± 2.43, 1.16 ± 0.85 for resistance at the occiput, C2 and C5 respectively (Fig. 2). The one-way ANOVA revealed a significant main effect for the location of resistance ($F = 5.04$; $P = 0.018$). The post-hoc SNK comparison showed significant differences between occiput versus C2 ($P = 0.024$) and C5 versus C2 ($P = 0.022$), but not between occiput versus C5 ($P = 0.625$) indicating that resistance at C2 resulted in the most selective activation of the semispinalis cervicis muscle relative to the splenius capitis.

4. Discussion

This study showed that manual resistance applied to the vertebral arch of C2 resulted in the most selective activation of the

semispinalis cervicis muscle (recorded at the level of C3) compared to resistance applied at the occiput or at the level of C5.

Studies examining the structure of the deep neck extensors show both fatty infiltration (Elliott et al., 2006) and atrophy (Elliott et al., 2008a) of the semispinalis cervicis muscle. Furthermore, the activity of the semispinalis cervicis muscle is reduced and less defined in patients with neck pain (Schomacher et al., 2011). Taken together, these findings suggest that exercises specifically activating the semispinalis cervicis are relevant to include within a training program for patients with neck pain. Despite this, very few investigations have examined whether specific exercises can selectively activate the deep cervical extensors.

A recent mfMRI study showed that an isometric head/neck extension at 20% of the maximum voluntary force performed in neutral position activated both the deep and superficial extensors equally in a group of healthy volunteers (Elliott et al., 2010). The same exercise performed in 15° of cranio-cervical extension

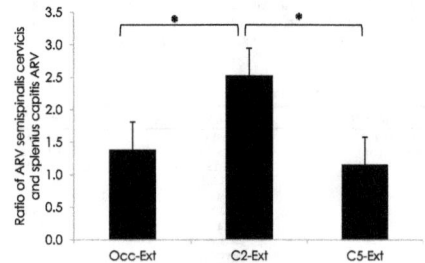

Fig. 2. Mean and standard error of the ratio of semispinalis cervicis and splenius capitis normalized EMG ARV during manual resistance applied at three different locations as the patients produced an extension force (*$P < 0.05$).

A Resistance at occiput   **B** Resistance at C2   **C** Resistance at C5

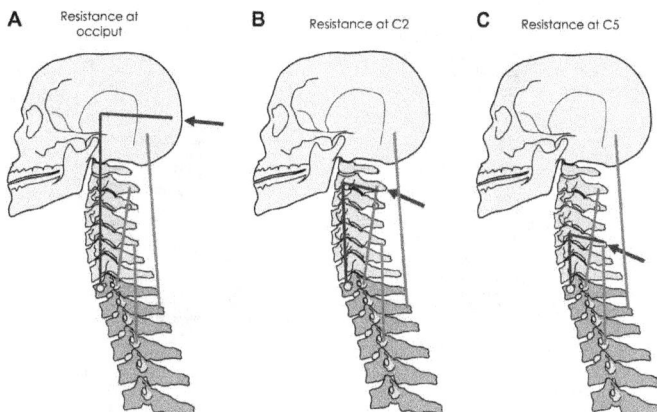

Fig. 3. Simplified illustration of the three manual resistances (dorsal arrows) with a common movement axis at segment C7-T1 and the assumption that other muscles stiffen all other spinal segments. The muscle fibres of the splenius capitis (representative fibre: dorsal line between T2 and occiput) are best suited to act on the angle lever of the occiput (A), while the muscle fibre of semispinalis cervicis inserting on C2 (representative fibre: ventral line from T1 to C2) acts best on the angle lever C2 (B) and the one inserting onto C5 (representative fibre: middle line between T4 and C5) on the angle lever of C5 (C). A similar analysis would be necessary for all other axis of rotation of the cervical spine for a comprehensive exploration of the system.

increased the activity of semispinalis capitis muscle compared to exercise performed in a neutral position, but not for the deep extensors below the level of C2 (Elliott et al., 2010). This is expected since multifidus and semispinalis cervicis have their highest attachments to the axis (C2) and are therefore not largely affected by cranio-cervical extension (Elliott et al., 2010). The findings of the present study also indicate that resistance to the occiput in a neutral position does not increase the activity of semispinalis cervicis relative to the splenius capitis.

When resistance was applied locally at C2 it resulted in the greatest activation of the semispinalis cervicis and the least activation of the splenius capitis. For home exercise, resistance by the therapist could be replaced by a theraband or a towel during the exercise. The observation that local resistance at C5 did not selectively activate the semispinalis cervicis may be related to the location of electrode placement. The fascicles of the semispinalis cervicis muscle originate from the transverse processes of the upper 5 or 6 thoracic vertebrae and insert on the cervical spinous processes, from the axis to the seventh cervical vertebrae inclusive. Each fascicle spans 4–6 segments (Schuenke et al., 2006; Drake et al., 2010). In this study we recorded activity of the semispinalis cervicis at the level of the third cervical vertebrae and therefore directly caudal to the location of resistance when applied at C2. A recent study has shown that synaptic input is distributed independently and non-uniformly to different fascicles of the semispinalis cervicis muscle and that motor units of the semispinalis cervicis are recruited according to the mechanical advantage of the muscle fibres (Schomacher et al., 2012). As illustrated in Fig. 3, fibres of the semispinalis cervicis inserting on C2 are better suited to resist an external force applied at C2. Splenius capitis and the fibres of semispinalis cervicis inserting below C2 require additional muscles to be active to stiffen the cervical spine in order to be able to resist the external force applied at C2.

A study investigating the relative cross-sectional area of the semispinalis cervicis in patients with whiplash-induced neck pain (Elliott et al., 2008a) showed significantly reduced muscle size in patients compared to controls but only at select levels of the spine (i.e. at C3, C5 and C6 only) suggesting that atrophy of the semispinalis cervicis muscle may vary between patients and spinal levels and could even be related to the location of the patients pain which is often at these levels (Bogduk and Marsland, 1988; Jull et al., 1988; Lord et al., 1996). This knowledge together with the results of the present study suggests that specific exercise/resistance should be applied to the segment closely above the site/s of dysfunction. However this should be confirmed in future studies.

4.1. Methodological considerations

A standardized intensity of manual resistance was not applied across conditions. This would have been difficult to measure and would not have been consistent with clinical practice, where the maximal resistance is adapted to the individual capabilities. Consequently the amount of force produced by the patients might have varied across conditions. However absolute values of EMG amplitude were not statistically compared but rather the ratio of EMG amplitude between the semispinalis cervicis and splenius capitis was assessed which should account for individual differences in the amount of resistance applied.

Due to the invasive nature of the experiment the number of participants was limited. For the same reason recordings were only performed unilaterally (on the side of greatest pain). Less invasive techniques such as muscle functional magnetic resonance imaging (Elliott et al., 2010) and tissue velocity ultrasound imaging (TVI) (Peolsson et al., 2010) may be useful in the future to examine a larger population to corroborate the present findings.

5. Conclusion

Patients with chronic neck pain are known to display reduced activity of the semispinalis cervicis muscle. The results of this study indicate that localized resistance can achieve relative isolation of the semispinalis cervicis muscle. This exercise approach may be relevant to include in the rehabilitation program for patients with neck pain. Future studies are needed to assess whether the activation of the semispinalis cervicis muscle can be increased with this exercise in patients with neck pain following a period of training and whether using this exercise approach offers pain relief.

References

Anderson JS, Hsu AW, Vasavada AN. Morphology, architecture, and biomechanics of human cervical multifidus. Spine 2005;30(4):E86–91.

Bexander CSM, Mellor R, Hodges PW. Effect of gaze direction on neck muscle activity during cervical rotation. Experimental Brain Research 2005;167:422–32.

Blouin J-S, Siegmund GP, Carpenter MG, Inglis JT. Neural control of superficial and deep neck muscles in humans. Journal of Neurophysiology 2007;98:920–8.

Bogduk N, Marsland A. The cervical zygapophysial joints as a source of neck pain. Spine 1988;13(6):610–7.

Bogduk N, McGuirk B. Management of acute and chronic neck pain, an evidence-based approach. Edinburgh: Elsevier; 2006.

Boyd-Clark LC, Briggs CA, Galea MP. Comparative histochemical composition of muscle fibres in a pre- and postvertebral muscle of the cervical spine. Journal of Anatomy 2001;199:709–16.

Drake RL, Vogl WA, Mitchell AWM. Gray's anatomy for students. 2nd ed. Philadelphia: Churchill Livingstone Elsevier; 2010.

Elliott JM, Jull G, Noteboom JT, Darnell R, Galloway G, Gibbon WW. Fatty infiltration in the cervical extensor muscles in persistent whiplash-associated disorders: a magnetic resonance imaging analysis. Spine 2006;31:E847–55.

Elliott JM, Jull G, Noteboom JT, Galloway G. MRI study of the cross-sectional area for the cervical musculature in patients with persistent whiplash associated disorders (WAD). Manual Therapy 2008a;13:258–65.

Elliott J, Sterling M, Noteboom JT, Darnell R, Galloway G, Jull G. Fatty infiltrate in the cervical extensor muscles is not a feature of chronic, insidious-onset neck pain. Clinical Radiology 2008b;63(6):681–7.

Elliott JM, O'Leary SP, Cagnie B, Durbridge G, Danneels L, Jull G. Craniocervical orientation affects muscle activation when exercising the cervical extensors in healthy subjects. Archives of Physical Medicine and Rehabilitation 2010;91:1418–22.

Falla D, Lindstrøm R, Rechter L, Farina D. Effect of pain on modulation in discharge rate of sternocleidomastoid motor units with force direction. Clinical Neurophysiology 2010;121(5):744–53.

Johnston V, Jull G, Souvlis T, Jimmieson N. Neck movement and muscle activity characteristics in female office workers with neck pain. Spine 2008;33(5):555–63.

Jull G, Bogduk N, Marsland AA. The accuracy of manual diagnosis for cervical zygapophysial joint pain syndromes. The Medical Journal of Australia 1988; 148(5):233–6.

Jull G, Sterling M, Falla D, Treleaven J, O'Leary S. Whiplash, headache, and neck pain: research-based directions for physical therapies. Edinburgh, Churchill Livingstone: Elsevier; 2008.

Kramer M, Schmid I, Sander S, Högel J, Eisele R, Kinzl L, et al. Guidelines for the intramuscular positioning of EMG electrodes in the semispinalis capitis and cervicis muscles. Journal of Electromyography and Kinesiology 2003;13:289–95.

Kristjansson E. Reliability of ultrasonography for the cervical multifidus muscle in asymptomatic and symptomatic subjects. Manual Therapy 2004;9:83–8.

Kumar S, Narayan Y, Prasad N, Shuaib A, Siddiqui ZA. Cervical electromyogram profile differences between patients of neck pain and control. Spine 2007; 32(8):E246–53.

Lee H, Nicholson LL, Adams RD. Neck muscle endurance, self-report, and range of motion data from subjects with treated and untreated neck pain. Journal of Manipulative and Physiological Therapeutics 2005;28:25–32.

Lee JP, Tseng WY, Shau YW, Wang CL, Wang HK, Wang SF. Measurement of segmental cervical multifidus contraction by ultrasonography in asymptomatic adults. Manual Therapy 2007;12:286–94.

Lindstrøm R, Schomacher J, Farina D, Rechter L, Falla D. Association between neck muscle coactivation, pain, and strength in women with neck pain. Manual Therapy 2011;16(1):80–6.

Lindstrøm R, Graven-Nielsen T, Falla D. Current pain and fear of pain contribute to reduced maximum voluntary contraction of neck muscles in patients with chronic neck pain. Archives of Physical Medicine and Rehabilitation; 2012. doi:10.1016/j.apmr.2012.04.014. Published ahead of print.

Lord S, Barnsley L, Wallis BJ, Bogduk N. Chronic cervical zygapophysial joint pain after whiplash. Spine 1996;21(15):1737–45.

Mayoux-Benhamou MA, Revel M, Vallee C. Selective electromyography of dorsal neck muscles in humans. Experimental Brain Research 1997;113:353–60.

O'Leary S, Falla D, Elliott JM, Jull G. Muscle dysfunction in cervical spine pain: implications for assessment and management. Journal of Orthopaedic & Sports Physical Therapy 2009;39(5):324–33.

O'Leary S, Cagnie B, Reeve A, Jull G, Elliott JM. Is there altered activity of the extensor muscles in chronic mechanical neck pain? A functional magnetic resonance imaging study. Archives of Physical Medicine and Rehabilitation 2011;92(6): 929–34.

Pearson AM, Ivancic PC, Ito S, Panjabi MM. Facet joint kinematics and injury mechanisms during simulated whiplash. Spine 2004;29:390–7.

Peolsson A, Brodin L-Å, Peolsson M. A tissue velocity ultrasound imaging investigation of the dorsal neck muscles during resisted isometric extension. Manual Therapy; 2010.

Prushansky T, Gepstein R, Gordon C, Dvir Z. Cervical muscles weakness in chronic whiplash patients. Clinical Biomechanics 2005;20:794–8.

Rankin G, Stokes M, Newham DJ. Size and shape of the posterior neck muscles measured by ultrasound imaging: normal values in males and females of different ages. Manual Therapy 2005;10:108–15.

Schomacher J, Farina D, Lindstroem R, Falla D. Chronic trauma-induced neck pain impairs the neural control of the deep semispinalis cervicis muscle. Clinical Neurophysiology; 2011. doi:10.1016/j.clinph.2011.11.033. Published ahead of print.

Schomacher J, Dideriksen JL, Farina D, Falla D. Recruitment of motor units in two fascicles of the semispinalis cervicis muscle. The Journal of Neurophysiology; 2012. doi:10.1152/jn.00953.2011. Published ahead of print.

Schuenke M, Schulte E, Schumacher U. Thieme atlas of anatomy, general anatomy and musculoskeletal system. Stuttgart – New York: Georg Thieme Verlag; 2006.

Sommerich CM, Joines SMB, Hermans V, Moon SD. Use of surface electromyography to estimate neck muscle activity. Journal of Electromyography and Kinesiology 2000;10:377–98.

Stokes M, Hides J, Elliott JM, Kiesel K, Hodges PW. Rehabilitative ultrasound imaging of the posterior paraspinal muscles. Journal of Orthopaedic & Sports Physical Therapy 2007;37(10):581–95.

Szeto GPY, Straker LM, O'Sullivan PB. A comparison of symptomatic and asymptomatic office workers performing monotonous keyboard work – 1: neck and shoulder muscle recruitment patterns. Manual Therapy 2005;10:270–80.

Vernon H, Mior S. The neck disability index: a study of reliability and validity. Journal of Manipulative and Physiological Therapeutics 1991;14(7):409–15.

Ylinen J. Physical exercises and functional rehabilitation for the management of chronic neck pain. Europa Medicophysica 2007;43:119–32.

About the author

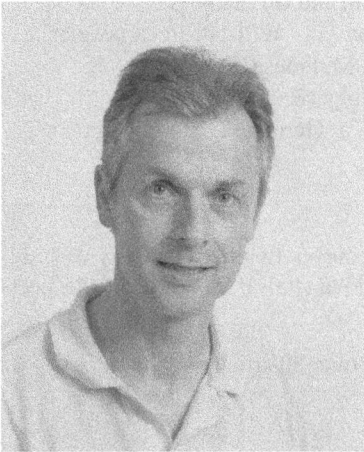

Jochen Schomacher, born 18.03.1961 (in Münster/Westf., Germany)
Address: Florastrasse 5, CH–8700 Küsnacht ZH, Switzerland

Diploma

2012	PhD in clinical science, Aalborg University, Denmark
2007	Master of Science in Physiotherapy (Germany: 90 ECTS)
2006	Bachelor of Science in Physiotherapy (Germany: 180 ECTS)
2002	Doctor of Physical Therapy (USA)
1998	National exam in Bobath therapy Concept (Germany)
1996	Instructor of Manual Therapy (OMT Kaltenborn-Evjenth Concept)
1996	State approved exam in M.C.M.K. (Moniteur Cadre en Masso-Kinésithérapie, France = Teacher and Cadre of Physiotherapy) (1 year fulltime study taken in 3 years)
1994	International exam in Orthopaedic Manipulative Therapy (IFOMPT)
1990	National exam in Manual Therapy (Germany)
1989	Staatl. anerkannter Krankengymnast (Physiotherapist)
1983	State approved exam as Therapist in Balneology (Staatl. anerkannter Kneipp- und med. Bademeister)

Professional career

Since 1996	Postgraduate freelance teacher of Manual Therapy
1992 - 2001	Teacher at a School of Physical Therapy (topics: Manual Therapy, Orthopedics, palpatory Anatomy, Medical Training Therapy, Biomecanics) in Germany
1989 – 1993	Practical work as physiotherapist in hospitals and privat practices in France, Switzerland and Germany
1986 – 1989	School of Physical Therapy in Willstätt-Eckartsweier (Germany, including 1 year in Mulhouse, France)
1983	School of Therapist in balneology (Bad Wörishofen)
1981 – 1985	Assistant in the practice of a German „natural doctor" (Heilpraktiker)

Actual functions

Instructor of Manual Therapy in postgraduate courses (mainly Germany & Italy) and at the Universities of Krems (Austria), Padova (Italy); co-editor of the peer-reviewed journal „Manuelle Therapie"

Publications: 2 books, some book chapters, and over 50 articles